Fundamentals of Cancer Chemotherapy

Fundamentals of Cancer Chemotherapy

Marion D. Cridland

Visiting Medical Officer, Royal Prince Alfred Hospital
and The Royal North Shore Hospital, Sydney

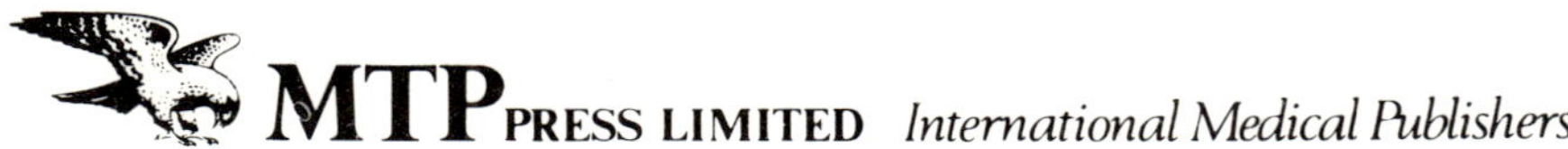

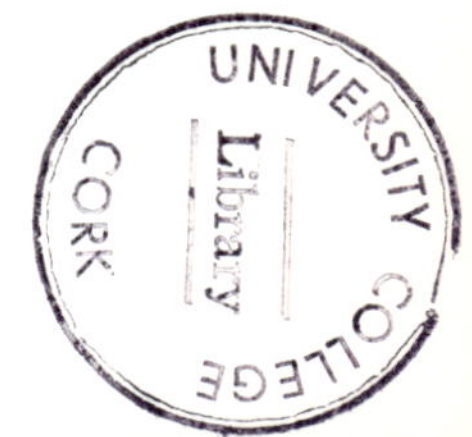

Fundamentals of Cancer Chemotherapy

Published in UK, Europe and Middle East
by MTP Press Limited
Falcon House
Lancaster
England

First Printing
ISBN 0-85200-508-3

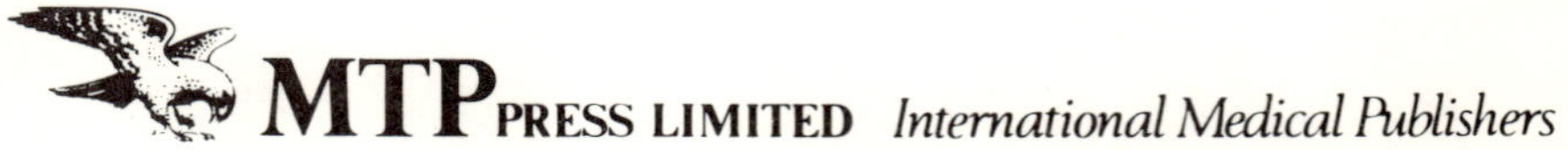

Printed at Bright Sun Printing Press Co. Ltd., Hong Kong.

Preface

Fundamentals of Cancer Chemotherapy has been written for medical students, postgraduate students in various fields, and for those practitioners unfamiliar with the chemotherapeutic management of malignant disease. With the increasing importance of cancer chemotherapy there is a need for most practitioners to acquaint themselves with this branch of therapeutics.

The book is not a treatment manual. Emphasis has been placed on general principles of treatment with little attention to the details of dosage and specific dose schedules. In the appendix are presented a few selected regimens in use at present, more for the purpose of illustration than practical application.

Marion D. Cridland
Sydney, 22nd May 1978

Contents

Chapter I

The Scope of Cancer Chemotherapy

The chemotherapy of malignant disease refers to the use of cytotoxic drugs. Hormones are also part of the drug treatment of some malignant conditions but they are not included in the term chemotherapy in this context. Corticosteroids, however, are used extensively in the management of some lymphomas and leukaemias and their application is necessarily considered in some detail here.

Cytotoxic drugs are general cellular poisons which have a deleterious effect, to a greater or lesser degree, on normal cells and a variety of tumours. Because these drugs are potentially lethal, cancer chemotherapy is largely a compromise between toxic and therapeutic effects and great care must be exercised in its use.

Excellent results tend to be limited to a few disorders, notably Hodgkin's disease, lymphocytic lymphomas, chronic leukaemia, acute lymphoblastic leukaemia of childhood, gestational choriocarcinoma and Burkitt's lymphoma. Good and sometimes exceptional results are also attainable in ovarian carcinoma, seminoma and histiocytic lymphoma. Good results are seen in myelomatosis, carcinoma of the breast and some soft tissue sarcomas. Chemotherapy may be a valuable adjunct to radiotherapy, Wilms' tumour being a case in particular: not only can the quality of life be greatly improved by chemotherapy but, in many instances survival time is prolonged, and in a few cases cure is achieved.

Unfortunately, in most malignant disease response is poor. Bronchogenic carcinoma, carcinoma of the pancreas, kidney and urinary tract, and others such as melanoma and osteogenic sarcoma are relatively resistant to chemotherapy. Most of the common carcinomas of the gastrointestinal tract also respond very poorly. Excellent results with chemotherapy in these forms of malignant disease are isolated triumphs.

Chemotherapy has probably been tried in every form of malignant disease, including the rarest, but not every one has received mention here. Not all the drugs in

current use have been described in the text, only better known examples from the various classes of cytotoxic agents. Some of the drugs have not yet been released for general use but have been included because their names appear from time to time in the medical journals.

Better results in recent years have been due more to improved methods of applying cytotoxic drugs than to the introduction of new drugs. However, in spite of improvements, drugs in current use are unlikely to achieve results in most common cancers comparable with those already seen in lymphomas for example. New approaches are clearly needed to overcome the present day inadequacies of cancer chemotherapy.

Chapter II

Historical Outline

In 1931, Adair and Bagg published the results of treatment with alcoholic solutions of mustard gas (dichlorodiethylsulphide). They referred to the observations of James Ewing and others on the destructive nature of burns caused by the gas and used it on tumours involving skin. It was applied topically in 12 cases and injected into the tumour in 1, a recurrent neurogenic sarcoma. The tumour regressed and remissions of a few months were obtained in other patients. Hopes were expressed for the future use of mustard gas in cases of localised disease.

In 1942, Goodman and Gilman were studying the pharmacology of nitrogen mustard derivatives (methylchloroethylamines) and noted their effects on lymphoid tissue and dividing cells. The two compounds which received attention were known by the code names HN2 and HN3, the latter, trichlorotriethylamine, being the first used clinically (Goodman et al., 1946). Clinical trials with HN2, mustine hydrochloride (nitrogen mustard, mechlorethamine hydrochloride), were initiated in 1943 in the United States and the results were reported by Rhoads in 1946.

Mustine and trichlorotriethylamine were parenteral alkylating agents. The first oral alkylating agent was tretamine (triethylenemelamine, TEM), and a series of oral nitrogen mustard derivatives was synthesised at the Chester Beatty Research Institute in London. Still widely used are the oral drugs chlorambucil, busulphan and melphalan which latter is also available for intravenous use.

Farber began clinical trials with folic acid antagonists in the 1940's, and methotrexate (amethopterin) emerged as the antimetabolite of choice (Farber et al., 1948). Purine analogues were also developed and the results with mercaptopurine (6-mercaptopurine) were published by Burchenal and others in 1953. The pyrimidine analogue fluorouracil (5-fluorouracil, 5-FU) went into clinical trials in 1958, and later thioguanine (6-thioguanine) and others were tried and introduced into clinical use.

Meanwhile, antibiotics were being investigated for antitumour properties. Actinomycin D (dactinomycin) from a strain of *Streptomyces* was shown to have antitumour activity in animals and early trials in 1956 showed promise (Farber, 1966). Almost at the same time mitomycin (mitomycin C) was developed in Japan.

The vinca alkaloids, vinblastine and vincristine were of special interest, being derived from a plant, the periwinkle *Vinca rosea*. Results of clinical trials demonstrating their value in Hodgkin's disease and other tumours were published in 1960 (Hodes et al., 1960; Johnson et al., 1960; Warwick et al., 1960).

The ability of some platinum complexes to inhibit cell division led to their investigation as anticancer drugs by Rosenberg and others. These compounds first underwent clinical trials in 1971, platinum diamminodichloride [*cis*-diammineplatinum (II)] being the one most extensively used so far (Gottlieb and Drewinko, 1975; Hill et al., 1975; Rosenberg, 1975).

Better methods of using cytotoxic agents have been developed in more recent times with guidelines from experimental models. In 1964 the simultaneous use of vincristine, methotrexate, mercaptopurine and prednisone, the so-called VAMP treatment, in acute lymphoblastic leukaemia of childhood led the way for combination chemotherapy in other forms of malignant disease (Freireich et al., 1964; Henderson, 1967; Henderson, 1969).

New cytotoxic drugs are sometimes received with undue enthusiasm when a more critical if not sceptical reception is more appropriate. The quest for new drugs continues with optimism and there is still great potential for the better application of available agents. However, unless ways are devised to reduce the adverse effects and to overcome the inherent drug resistance of the common cancers, drugs in current use will remain an unsatisfactory form of treatment.

Chapter III

Pharmacology and Mode of Action of Cytotoxic Drugs

1. Cytotoxic Effects

1.1 Alkylating Agents

Alkylating agents comprise a wide variety of compounds with different physicochemical properties. They include, among others, the nitrogen and sulphur mustards, sulphonates, alkyl halides, diazo compounds, epoxides, and the lactones. Thousands of alkylating agents have been synthesised but, after appropriate screening tests, only a few have been submitted for clinical trial. As well as having a firm place in cancer chemotherapy, agents of this type are used as solvents and fumigants in a number of industrial processes and for sterilisation of insect pests.

Alkylating agents have in common the property of undergoing chemical reactions resulting in the formation of covalent linkages (alkylation). The alkyl groups have an affinity for the DNA molecule (predominantly the 7 nitrogen in the purine base, guanine), and exert their effect by distorting the double helix. Thus replication is disrupted (Price, 1968; Price et al., 1969).

The nitrosoureas, carmustine (BCNU), lomustine (CCNU) and semustine (methyl-CCNU) owe their activity to alkylation and also to inhibition of enzymes concerned with DNA synthesis. They pass into the cell, probably by passive diffusion. There the nitrosoureas undergo decomposition into chloroethyl carbonium ions which react with nucleic acids by alkylation, and into isocyanates which interact with amino acids and proteins. Being lipophilic they reach higher concentrations in the brain compared with the water soluble agents. They are effective against èxperimental rat brain sarcomas and implanted intracranial L1210 leukaemia in mice. They are also most effective against other types of tumour in animals (Burchenal and Carter, 1972; Carter, 1973).

Early studies of alkylating agents demonstrated their selective action on lymphoid tissue, bone marrow, intestinal mucosa and lymphoid tumours (Elson, 1958; Smith et al., 1958; Steinberg et al., 1958). Depletion of lymph nodes and spleen, together with bone marrow aplasia, are characteristic changes produced by all the alkylating agents. However, there is no selective concentration of the drugs in those tissues showing the most severe injury: at a subcellular level they are distributed in the mitochondrial, microsomal and nuclear fractions of resistant as well as sensitive cells. They used to be called radiomimetic drugs as they produced biological effects similar to those resulting from ionizing radiation; however, there are profound differences between the chemical lesions caused by these agents and the damage caused by radiation.

A list of some of the more commonly used alkylating agents is shown in table I.

Absorption from the gastrointestinal tract is satisfactory but may be variable. A dose of most alkylating agents disappears rapidly from the blood, is taken up by the tissues and is immediately fixed. In the case of cyclophosphamide, the drug is first converted to its active form by microsomal enzymes. There is wastage of course, from combination with serum proteins and tissues other than target cells. The reaction products of the alkylating agents are metabolised and excreted by the kidney over several days.

Some alkylating agents are oral preparations, others are parenteral, and the mode of administration desired may influence the choice of drug. Nitrogen mustard is available only as a parenteral preparation which tends to sclerose the tissues; thiotepa (triethylene thiophosphoramide) is also a parenteral alkylating agent. Chlorambucil and busulphan are both oral drugs while melphalan and cyclophosphamide are available for oral and intravenous or localised use.

The alkylating agents are the most widely used cytotoxic drugs either alone or in combination with other classes. They are the basic drugs of choice in the chemotherapy of Hodgkin's disease, lymphomas, chronic leukaemias, myeloma, myeloproliferative disorders, ovarian carcinoma and seminoma and a number of less sensitive malignant diseases (Ochoa, 1969). They are also used as 'immunosuppressive' agents in non-malignant conditions. Cyclophosphamide is the only alkylating agent used regularly in acute leukaemia, and the others are yet to undergo adequate clinical trial (Fernbach et al., 1960). The results of the treatment of brain tumours in man with carmustine and lomustine are less impressive than those in animals. The nitrosoureas are nevertheless more useful than other cytotoxic drugs in the treatment of brain tumours. The nitrosoureas are active against Hodgkin's disease and they are included in several combined regimens for lymphomas, bronchogenic carcinoma, carcinoma of the gastrointestinal tract and others.

In general, all the alkylating agents have much the same range of activity and usually there is little point in changing from one to another when a tumour fails to respond. Claims for the superiority of one alkylating agent over another are sometimes made, but differences in dose, dose schedule and mode of administration tend to

Table I. Classes and examples of cancer chemotherapy drugs

Class	Example	Synonyms	Proprietary name
Alkylating agents	Busulphan		'Myleran'
	Carmustine	BCNU	'BiCNU'
	Chlorambucil		'Leukeran'
	Cyclophosphamide		'Endoxan', 'Endoxana', 'Endoxan Asta'
	Lomustine	CCNU	
	Melphalan	Phenylalanine nitrogen mustard	'Alkeran'
	Mitobronitol	Dibromomannitol, DBM	'Myelobromol'
	Mustine hydrochloride	Chlorethazine hydrochloride, nitrogen mustard, HN2.	'Mustargen Hydrochloride'
	Semustine	Methyl-CCNU, methyl lomustine	
	Thiotepa	Triethylene thiophosphoramide	'Thio-Tepa'
	Tretamine	Triethylene melamine, TEM	
Antimetabolites	Azathioprine		'Imuran'
	Cytarabine	Cytosine arabinoside, ara-C	'Cytosar'
	Fluorouracil	5-Fluorouracil, 5-FU	'Fluoro-uracil', 'Efudix Cream', 'Fluoroplex Cream'
	Mercaptopurine	6-Mercaptopurine, 6-MP	'Puri-Nethol'
	Methotrexate	Amethopterin, MXT	'Methotrexate'
	Thioguanine	6-Thioguanine, 6-TG	'Lanvis'
Antibiotics	Actinomycin D	Dactinomycin	'Cosmegen', 'Lyovac'
	Bleomycin	Bleomycin sulphate	'Bleomycin'
	Daunorubicin	Daunomycin, rubidomycin	'Cerubidin'
	Doxorubicin	Adriamycin	'Adriamycin'
	Mithramycin		'Mithracin'
	Mitomycin	Mitomycin C	'Mitomycin C'
	Streptozocin	Streptozotocin	
Miscellaneous	Colaspase	Asparaginase, L-asparaginase	'Crasnitin'
	Dacarbazine	DTIC	'DTIC-Dome'
	Hydroxyurea	Hydroxycarbamide	'Hydrea'
	Platinum diamminodichloride	Cis-platinum, *cis*-diammineplatinum (II), DDP	
	Procarbazine		'Natulan'
	Vinblastine	Vincaleucoblastine	'Velbe'
	Vincristine	Leurocristine	'Oncovin'

invalidate comparisons. However, because the route of administration or the dose schedule can influence response, a trial of a second alkylating agent, or the same one in a different form, may be warranted if the initial response is not satisfactory. For example, a change from oral chlorambucil to a single large intravenous dose of mustine may prove better, just as a change from oral to intravenous cyclophosphamide may prove more effective.

Certainly side effects can differ among alkylating agents although some of these could be due to degradation products and not to the alkylating component. However, some experimental studies have suggested possible differences between alkylating agents that might have some clinical significance. Mustine seems the most non-specific cell toxin and cyclophosphamide the most selective, though reports vary depending on the conditions of the experiment. Busulphan is also somewhat different from others of the group in having more delayed effects and more readily causing thrombocytopenia. Nevertheless, the similarities of the alkylating agents are more striking than their differences and, whatever the differences might be under experimental conditions, they do not appear to be great clinically.

The mutagenic effects of alkylating agents were recognised early and those popular experimental tools, *drosophila,* were among the first to undergo mutation induced by alkylating agents (Auerbach, 1958).

The carcinogenic potential of alkylating agents was investigated in experimental animals by Haddow and others during the early years of cancer chemotherapy (Haddow, 1953). Compared with the incidence in animals, cytotoxic drug induced carcinogenesis appears to be rare in man. Carcinoma of the bladder has been reported after treatment with cyclophosphamide and the reported incidence of acute leukaemia is increasing. It remains speculative whether such cases result from a direct carcinogenic effect, or from immunosuppression, or are only a chance association. There is evidence to support the concept that normal immune mechanisms play a part in preventing malignant change. Lymphoid cells, T cells in particular, are those predominantly involved. There is a greater incidence of malignant disease in immunodeficient states, and also among renal transplant recipients and other patients immunosuppressed with long term corticosteroids and azathioprine, mercaptopurine or cyclophosphamide. A direct carcinogenic effect should be distinguished from malignant change resulting from immunosuppression, although a defect in immune surveillance could perhaps permit expression of any carcinogenic propensity a cytotoxic drug might have.

Adverse effects on the developing embryo were expected, and studied in considerable detail, establishing that alkylating agents can produce gross fetal malformation in animals (Di Paolo, 1969; Murphy et al., 1958). The dysmorphogenic effects are dose dependent but differ in some respects from one animal to another, largely because of differences in experimental design. Such additional factors as solubility, and thus transport across the placenta, probably account for some of the observed differences. In the human, the 3rd to 8th week of embryonic development is the most critical period, but the risk of malformation in the human embryo is very much less than in experimental animals.

The effect on the gonads, especially spermatogenesis, has been well described and is directly cytotoxic (Miller, 1971; Richter et al., 1960). The possibility of mutagenic change within the gonads should discourage parenthood.

The mode of action of alkylating agents with respect to carcinogenesis, mutagenesis and dysmorphogenesis has not yet been clarified. Some potent mutagens are not dysmorphogenic or carcinogenic. Alkylation might be involved or the effects might be due to metabolites of the drugs (Malling and de Serres, 1969).

1.2 Antimetabolites

Antimetabolites interfere with metabolic pathways, particularly those involved in nucleic acid synthesis.

Methotrexate is a folic acid antagonist which binds to dihydrofolate reductase to prevent the conversion of folic to tetrafolic acid. This deprivation interferes with the folate dependent utilisation of one-carbon compounds for *de novo* synthesis of nucleic acid.

Methotrexate is available for oral and parenteral use. After an intravenous injection of methotrexate, there is rapid uptake by most tissues. Very little reaches the CSF. Some of the drug excreted in bile is reabsorbed from the small intestine and metabolites of methotrexate are reabsorbed from the large intestine. It is excreted by the kidney by a mechanism involving active renal tubular secretion and renal function should be checked before the drug is given (Condit, 1971; Oliverio and Zaharko, 1971).

Cytarabine (cytosine arabinoside), mercaptopurine and fluorouracil are analogues of the metabolites deoxycytidine, hypoxanthine and uracil respectively. Cytarabine is first phosphorylated to its triphosphate form and inhibits DNA polymerase. It is rapidly deaminated to uracil arabinoside and excreted in the urine. The thioprine mercaptopurine is converted to its nucleotide 6-thioinosinic acid. As a purine antagonist, it is incorporated into DNA and RNA and also interferes with an early stage of *de novo* synthesis of purines. Azathioprine is an imidazole derivative of mercaptopurine and is converted to mercaptopurine *in vivo*. It has been suggested that the imidazole component of azathioprine contributes to its effectiveness as an immunosuppressive drug. At a cellular level, mercaptopurine and azathioprine tend to have a preferential effect on T lymphocytes. The pyrimidine fluorouracil is also converted to its active nucleotide form, 5-fluorodeoxyuridylic acid which inhibits thymidylate synthetase, an enzyme required in the *de novo* synthesis of thymidine. All these antagonists are readily metabolised, either completely or incompletely, then excreted in urine or bile.

The antimetabolites were previously used mainly in acute leukaemia but their use has now been extended to most forms of malignant disease. Some are also used as immunosuppressive drugs. Methotrexate, as well as being of value in acute leukaemia either alone or in combination, also has activity against choriocarcinoma, carcinoma of the breast and ovary, a few soft tissue sarcomas, teratoma and several others. It is also given to suppress the proliferative activity of psoriasis (Weinstein, 1971). Methotrexate is sometimes given in very high doses with so-called folinic acid 'rescue'. Folinic acid is the antidote to methotrexate and if given within the appropriate time interval after the administration of methotrexate, can prevent or reduce the toxic side effects (Douglas and Price, 1973; Goldie et al., 1972). This method operates successfully when differences between the growth kinetics of tumour and normal cells are suitable; folinic acid would otherwise rescue malignant cells as well.

Colorectal carcinoma is known to respond to fluorouracil. It is active in about 30% of cases of ovarian carcinoma and is frequently included in combined schedules, especially for carcinoma of the breast.

Like the alkylating agents the antimetabolites, and probably all the cytotoxic drugs, are potentially dangerous to the developing embryo and to the gonads. Methotrexate in particular has a reputation for causing fetal abnormalities, deformities of the face being a striking feature (Powell and Ekert, 1971).

1.3 Antibiotics

Some of the antibiotics with anticancer activity are listed in table I. Most are derived from strains of *Streptomyces* and their effects are exerted mainly through inhibition of DNA synthesis. Their precise modes of action are incompletely understood.

Actinomycin D inhibits DNA directed RNA synthesis. Daunorubicin and adriamycin (doxorubicin) bind to DNA, and bleomycin inhibits cell division in a similar way. Alkylation might be involved in the action of mitomycin (mitomycin C) [Cohen et al., 1976; Cox and Farmer, 1977].

Antibiotics and their metabolites can be detected in most tissues after administration; they are excreted mainly in urine. Daunorubicin and adriamycin and their metabolites, and some unchanged actinomycin D, are also excreted to a significant extent in bile.

The antibiotics figure prominently in the chemotherapy of acute leukaemia, but one, actinomycin D was established years ago as a useful drug in Wilms' tumour and is of some value in testicular tumours. Daunorubicin and adriamycin are used in conditions other than acute leukaemia, and adriamycin in particular has been tried with appreciable success in Hodgkin's disease, lymphomas and several carcinomas. Bleomycin has some effect on squamous cell carcinoma of the head and neck and on several other tumours. It is more often used in combination with other drugs (Bull et al., 1972; Gray and Michaels, 1972; Halnan et al., 1972; Mathe et al., 1970).

1.4 Vinca Alkaloids

Vinblastine and vincristine are alkaloids extracted from the plant *Vinca rosea*. They cause cell death in metaphase by disrupting cellular microtubules, a component of the mitotic spindle. *In vitro* in certain concentrations they prevent the uptake of thymidine into DNA and uridine into RNA and can block protein synthesis. Their degradation products are excreted in bile.

In spite of their similar chemical structure and *in vitro* activity, vinblastine and vincristine have somewhat different clinical effects and toxicity. Most of these differences are probably more a matter of degree than of specific characteristics. Vincristine is of notable value in acute lymphoblastic leukaemia and is less myelosuppressive than vinblastine. They both have a wide range of activity, comparable with the alkylating agents, which includes lymphomas, Hodgkin's disease, carcinoma of the breast and ovary, choriocarcinoma and many others (Carbone et al., 1963; Hodes et al., 1962; Hill and Loeb, 1961; Marmont and Damasio, 1967; Warwick et al., 1960).

1.5 Procarbazine

Procarbazine, a methylhydrazine derivative, breaks down DNA *in vitro* and seems to act like an alkylating agent having a similar spectrum of activity. It is used mainly in combination chemotherapy in Hodgkin's disease and lymphomas. Most of it is broken down and excreted, principally in the urine (Spiers, 1967).

1.6 Hydroxyurea

Hydroxyurea interferes with the production of deoxynucleotides for DNA synthesis, for instance by preventing reduction of cytidine to deoxycytidine. It also inhibits incorporation of thymidine into DNA but has no inhibitory effect on RNA or protein synthesis.

Hydroxyurea has a place in the treatment of late stage chronic myelocytic leukaemia when busulphan is no longer effective (Kennedy and Yarbro, 1966).

1.7 Asparaginase

Unique among chemotherapeutic drugs asparaginase (colaspase) is an enzyme. It breaks down asparagine and those tumour cells which lack asparagine synthetase are thus deprived of their exogenous source of asparagine. It does not cause bone marrow depression but has toxic effects on the liver and other organs. It is of some value in

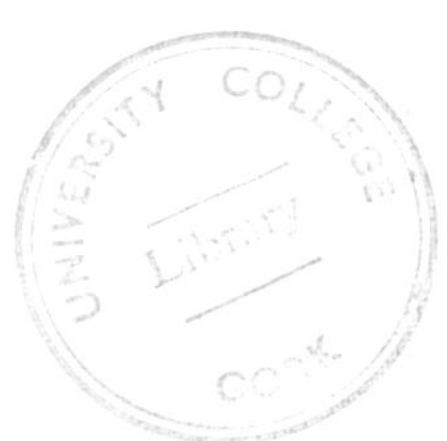

acute leukaemia and is usually given in combination with other drugs (Burchenal and Karnofsky, 1970; Cohen et al., 1976; Editorial, 1971).

1.8 Dacarbazine

Dacarbazine (Dimethyl-triazeno-imidazole carboxamide, DTIC) is an analogue of the precursor amino imidazole carboxamide in *de novo* purine synthesis. It is activated by N-demethylation in the liver to liberate the precursor and an alkylating component. Its degradation products are excreted in the urine.

Dacarbazine is of interest because a number of studies have shown it to have some effect against melanoma. It is also active in Hodgkin's disease, lymphocytic lymphoma and, to a lesser extent, in soft tissue sarcomas (Cohen et al., 1976).

1.9 Platinum Coordination Complexes

Platinum diamminodichloride (*cis*-diammineplatinum [II], cis-platinum) has been the most extensively tested, being highly effective against a number of experimental tumours in mice and rats, and the first submitted for clinical trial (Rosenberg, 1975).

At low concentrations the drug inhibits DNA synthesis without interfering with the synthesis of precursors and without significant effect on RNA or protein synthesis. These initial observations suggested a direct interaction with DNA.

The platinum complexes passively diffuse into the cell where hydrolysis of the chloride groups occurs, leaving two active sites to combine with nuclear DNA. The higher chloride concentration outside the cell limits hydrolysis of the complexes in the body fluids.

It has also been noted that platinum complexes depress virally coded information in bacteria. It is suggested that the reaction might enhance the antigenicity of a tumour which might explain the rapid regression of some advanced transplanted tumours in animals treated with these compounds.

Platinum diamminodichloride is given intravenously and is distributed through all tissues, with higher concentrations found in liver and kidney. Most of the platinum is excreted by the kidney within 48 hours.

Like most other cytotoxic drugs, the platinum coordination complexes cause nausea, vomiting, bone marrow depression and immunosuppression. They also cause renal tubular necrosis and probably damage to the cochlea. These selective side effects on renal and acoustic function are usually dose related, cumulative and irreversible.

Platinum diamminodichloride has a similar range of activity to that of the alkylating agents but might be more active in squamous carcinoma of the head and neck. It has produced most encouraging results in testicular tumours and is useful in ovarian carcinoma (Gottlieb and Drewinko, 1975; Hill et al., 1975).

2. Immunosuppressive Effects

Cytotoxic drugs and corticosteroids are immunosuppressive, a feature which is utilised with varying success in diseases in which immune responses are pathological or have pathological consequences (Gerber and Steinberg, 1976; Skinner and Schwartz, 1972).

Their exact mode of action in this regard is poorly understood. The drugs affect the function of B and T lymphocytes to greater or lesser extent so that humoral and cell mediated immunity may be suppressed. Anticancer drugs also have anti-inflammatory action which might account for part of their therapeutic effect in some conditions.

Of the alkylating agents, cyclophosphamide has been the most extensively investigated and used for immunosuppression. It is not necessarily the alkylating agent of choice, in fact its side effects create problems. Cyclophosphamide inhibits proliferating cells including antigen stimulated cells. It alters both B and T cell function but in high doses has a more preferential action on B cells, perhaps because of their greater metabolic activity.

Azathioprine and mercaptopurine have a preferential effect on T lymphocytes, consistent with the effectiveness of these drugs in the maintenance of renal transplants. Why these drugs should affect cell mediated immunity with little if any suppression of antibody production by B cells is obscure. Methotrexate can interfere with antibody production, and in animals has been shown to suppress the homograft reaction. Methotrexate is unsuitable for use in kidney transplant cases because of its toxicity when renal function is impaired (Thomas & Storb, 1971).

Information on the mode of action of corticosteroids is fragmentary. Corticosteroids are lymphocytolytic but the specific series of events leading to lymphocytolysis has not been clearly defined. Steroids have been shown to affect cellular metabolism, DNA and protein synthesis and to interfere with the processing of antigen. The effect on B cells may be largely indirect by preventing differentiation of precursors into antibody forming cells.

Sensitised T lymphocytes are particularly sensitive to corticosteroids which accounts in part for the value of steroids in transplant cases. Their anti-inflammatory effect however could be the more important component in the suppression of the graft versus host reaction.

3. Conclusions

With few exceptions cytotoxic drugs act primarily by interfering with the synthesis or function of DNA. They are general cellular poisons damaging normal as well as malignant cells.

Alkylating agents combine with nucleic acids. Mustine, its derivatives and other similarly reactive compounds, are used extensively in cancer chemotherapy.

Antimetabolites interfere with metabolic pathways in the synthesis of nucleic acids. They are well established in the treatment of acute leukaemia and are also active against many other malignant tumours.

Antibiotics with anticancer activity inhibit DNA synthesis. Most are useful in acute leukaemia but also have a place in the treatment of many other conditions.

The vinca alkaloids cause cell death in metaphase and interfere with DNA and RNA synthesis. Their range of activity is similar to that of alkylating agents. Compounds such as procarbazine, hydroxyurea and others are also inhibitors of DNA synthesis.

Cytotoxic drugs are immunosuppressive, affecting humoral as well as cell mediate immunity.

Chapter IV

Cytokinetics and the Cell Cycle

Experimental evaluation of anticancer agents on L1210 mouse leukaemia by Skipper and co-workers (Skipper et al., 1964; Skipper et al., 1965) revealed several important fundamental facts of clinical relevance:

1) A dose of a cytotoxic agent will kill a constant fraction, not a constant number, of cells; that is, it will kill say, 95% or 99% whether 100 million or 100 cells are present.

2) There is a close relationship between dosage level and the percentage of a given leukaemic cell population killed by an effective drug, and the higher the dose the greater the chance of killing all the malignant cells.

3) At least the greater part of the surviving fraction of cells is a proliferating population and there is no hope of cure while this fraction continues to proliferate and compensate for those killed.

4) The average life span of the mouse is consistently related to the size of the leukaemic inoculum and the chances of eradicating all the malignant cells is greatest when the number is small.

The mouse leukaemia L1210 experimental system is a uniform, predictable malignant cell population. Skipper emphasised that the work set out to seek 'basic knowledge' and did not necessarily imply that the information was applicable to cancer chemotherapy in man, even in the treatment of acute leukaemia. Unfortunately by the time a malignant disease is clinically evident, the tumour load is already enormous. Also the use of high dosage is limited by the adverse effects on normal cells. Nevertheless, the basic knowledge obtained, though not to be transposed too literally to the clinical scene, holds true in principle and provided guidelines for dose schedules in the treatment of human disease. The essential clinical guidelines that emerged suggested that treatment should be more successful when the tumour load was small and that high dose short term schedules had an advantage over long term low dose schedules.

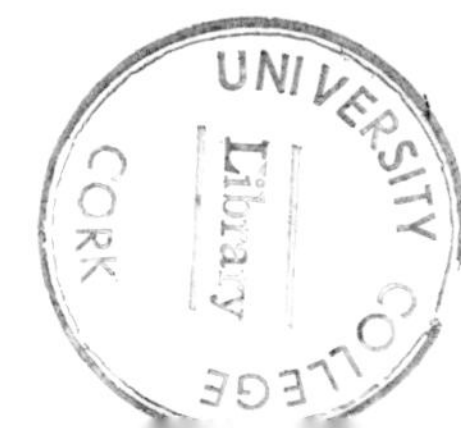

Skipper and his colleagues raised the possibility that the constant fractional survival of cells was due to their noncycling stage at the time of exposure to the drugs. The significance of the cell cycle in relation to cancer treatment was explored by Bruce et al., (1966).

The cell cycle is the interval between the midpoint of one mitosis and the next in the daughter cells. After the M phase or mitosis, there is the G_1 interphase. Thereafter is the S or DNA synthetic phase and another interphase, G_2 (fig. 1). Cells not actively engaged in division are said to be resting in the G_0 state from which they can be stimulated to cycle again. Cells that leave the cycle permanently, die without further dividing.

Cells are further subdivided into two compartments, stem cells which regenerate stem cells that are responsible for the continuing survival of a cell population, and non-stem cells destined for differentiation. The existence of malignant stem cells awaits proof but clearly their elimination is essential if chemotherapy is to effect a cure. Preservation of normal stem cells is essential for the survival of the patient.

Bruce and his co-workers (Bruce et al., 1966) developed a quantitative method for measuring the effect of cytotoxic drugs on the survival of normal haemopoietic and transplanted lymphoma colony-forming cells in the mouse. Cell suspensions of mouse haemopoietic stem cells and lymphoma cells from the spontaneous mouse lymphoma were injected into animals and the number of colonies formed were counted after treatment with anticancer drugs. The effects were assayed by the extent of their inhibition of colony formation by the normal cells and the rapidly dividing lymphoma cells. From these initial studies cytotoxic drugs were classified according to their site of action or effect upon the cell cycle, namely non-specific, phase-specific and cycle-specific (table II).

The action was called non-specific when it equally affected resting as well as proliferating cells. Radiation and high doses of mustine can produce non-specific effects. The survival curves decreased exponentially with increasing doses whether given as a single dose or in divided doses over 24 hours, and the dose curves were similar for lymphoma and the slower dividing normal cells. These findings indicated the action was not dependent on the proliferative state of the exposed cells.

Drugs sparing cells in G_0 but causing cell death during a particular phase of the cell cycle were called phase-specific. In this case survival curves decreased exponentially to a minimum with increasing dose, with little further cell kill at higher doses of the drug, provided the exposure time was short. The response to a dose of a phase-specific drug depended on the proportion of cells in that phase at the time. A lethal dose for the cells therefore killed only that fraction. In the experimental model cytotoxic agents of this type effected a differential kill, with 20 to 60% of normal cells surviving while only 0.06 to 0.08% of lymphoma cells survived. Many of the agents originally classified as phase-specific have since been shown to affect more than one phase of the cycle but to different degrees. Drugs classified as phase-specific include cytarabine, hydroxyurea, methotrexate, vinblastine and vincristine.

Cycle-specific drugs kill cells throughout the cell cycle and to some extent spare resting cells in G_0. In the experimental model, cell survival decreased exponentially with increasing dose and the lymphoma cells were 6 to 10 times more sensitive than haemopoietic stem cells. Unlike the effect with the phase-specific drugs, there was no saturation value for the dose survival curve at higher doses. Examples of cycle-specific drugs are mustine, chlorambucil, melphalan, cyclophosphamide, busulphan, thiotepa, the nitrosoureas, daunorubicin, adriamycin, fluorouracil and actinomycin D.

The differential sensitivity to cycle-or phase-specific agents in Bruce's model depended primarily upon the difference in the rate of proliferation of the two cell types and upon the proportion proliferating. The few lymphoma cells surviving were presumed to be those not passing through the generation cycle during the period of treatment. In contrast, a much greater proportion of normal haemopoietic cells were in the non-proliferative state of G_0. Rapidly dividing cells are more vulnerable not only because they are progressing through the cell cycle but also because there is less time for repair processes that might overcome the effect of the cytotoxic drugs.

Malignant cells do not necessarily proliferate more rapidly, in fact their average generation time can be longer than that of most normal cells. The therapeutic advantage can be gained when there is a fortuitous difference between the proliferative activity of the normal and malignant cell population. If the growth fraction is large then a relatively greater proportion of that cell population will be exposed to the drug. Under clinical conditions it is not known what proportion of a malignant cell popula-

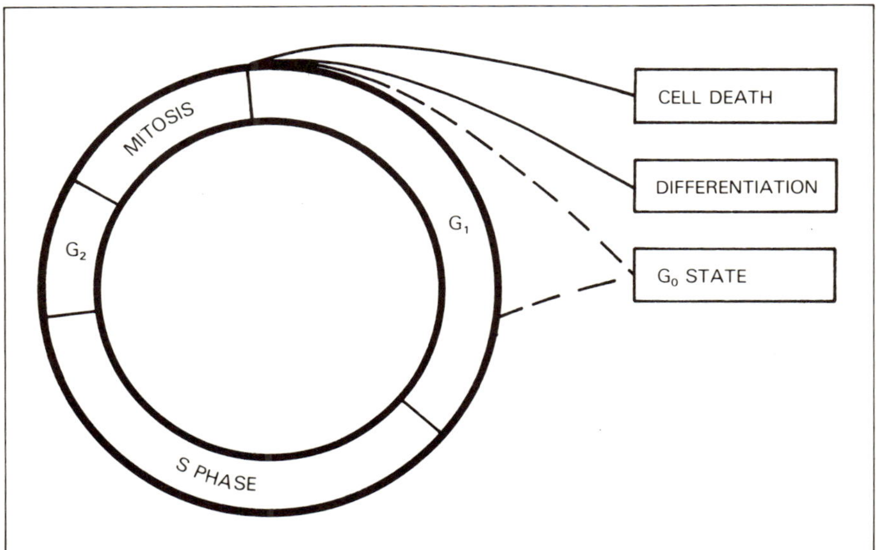

Fig. 1. The cell cycle.

Table II. Types of cytotoxic activity of chemotherapeutic agents in mouse lymphoma model (after Bruce et al., 1966)

Class	Cytotoxic activity	Example
Non-specific	Proliferating and resting cells killed	Mustine (high dose)
Phase-specific	Proliferating cells killed in certain phases of the cycle only	Cytarabine Hydroxyurea Methotrexate Vinblastine Vincristine
Cycle-specific	Proliferating cells killed throughout the cell cycle	Actinomycin D Adriamycin Busulphan Chlorambucil Cyclophosphamide Daunorubicin Fluorouracil Melphalan Mustine Thiotepa Nitrosoureas

tion is proliferating, inherently resistant to the drug, or partially protected in G_0 state, nor is it known what fraction of the proliferating population has been eliminated and to what extent the stem cell population has been affected. Available data on the growth kinetics of solid tumours indicate a range of 20 to 70% in the growth fraction which means that some 30 to 80% of cells are not actively dividing and are hence not particularly vulnerable to cytotoxic drugs. The doubling time of solid tumours may range from a week to a year or more and there is a wide range of variation even within the one tumour type (Berenbaum, 1969; Friedman et al., 1972; Hill and Baserga, 1975; Hryniuk and Bertino, 1971; Rosenoer and Curby, 1975).

A few figures drawn from the work of Killmann (1972) and others on human leukaemic blast cells illustrate the complexities of the problem of designing appropriately precise dose schedules in the treatment of acute leukaemia. At the time of diagnosis it was estimated that 15 to 35% of the blast cells in the bone marrow were actively proliferating. The generation time of these cells was usually about 50 to 60 hours but varied from 45 to 84 hours. Normal myeloblasts averaged 15 hours, promyelocytes 24 hours and myelocytes 51 hours. The turnover time for slowly proliferating blast cells ranged from 2 days to 2 weeks. There was wide variation in the duration of the various phases of the cell cycle and variation in the number of cells in a particular phase at any given time. Some 4 to 14% of leukaemic myeloblasts were found to be engaged in DNA synthesis compared with 40 to 70% of normal cells. The S phase varied from 15 to 20 hours or longer for leukaemic cells, with a normal S phase of 13 to 14 hours. The average time of mitosis in leukaemic and normal blast cells was 60 minutes and 30 minutes respectively. Finally, the duration of G_1 was subject to wide variation.

In the isolated systems of experimental models, the cells are relatively uniform in type and behaviour, which is not the case in malignant disease of man. Quantitative data on the effects of drugs on experimental systems are more readily obtained, mitotic intervals can be measured and cycles synchronised so that the maximum number of cells are vulnerable at the same time. Tumours in man do not consist of homogeneous populations of cells but of heterogeneous groups. In a given cell population in human disease there is no uniformity in the duration of cell phases or the cycle time. It is variable and not synchronised. While synchronisation of cell cycles can be achieved experimentally it is not surprising that attempts have met with little success clinically. To synchronise the cycles or recruit malignant cells from a resting state must also involve vulnerable normal cells and might thereby increase the toxic side effects.

Basic information from experimental models has guided the clinician towards a far better compromise between the toxic and therapeutic effects of cancer chemotherapy. The drugs certainly can act selectively against malignant cells in some malignant diseases of humans, however, even in the most sensitive of conditions the drugs must be administered with care. While the similarities between man and mouse may be striking, their malignant diseases are dissimilar. In man it cannot be assumed that most normal cells are safely resting in the G_0 state while most of the malignant cells are conveniently cycling. Pancytopenia with recovery of the tumour is a much more common event than cure by chemotherapy.

Conclusions

Cytotoxic drugs kill a constant fraction of a given cell population. Only those cells actively proliferating are especially vulnerable. In general, short term high dose chemotherapy is the most effective.

Drugs may be classified according to their predominant effect on the cell cycle: cycle-specific drugs can destroy cells throughout the generation cycle; phase-specific drugs affect one or more phases of the cycle, sparing resting cells.

The greater the proportion of sensitive cells actively cycling, the greater the chance of reducing the cell population. The chances of killing all the cells are greatest when the cell population is small.

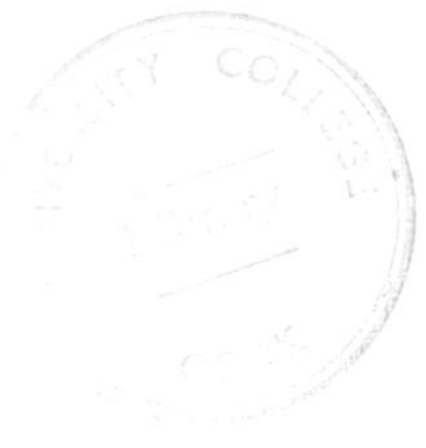

Chapter V

Adverse Effects and Complications of Treatment

The greatest single hazard in cancer chemotherapy is damage to haemopoietic tissue and the resultant complications. In general, the adverse haematological effects are similar with all the offending drugs. There are a few differences such as delayed bone marrow depression that can occur with the nitrosoureas and busulphan and a greater tendency to cause thrombocytopenia is another feature that these drugs have in common. Vincristine on the other hand, is less likely to affect megakaryocytes. Megaloblastic anaemia is predictably a side effect of methotrexate but has been reported after use of the nitrosoureas.

In the general management of patients with Hodgkin's disease, lymphomas, ovarian carcinoma, chronic leukaemias and many others, treatment rarely causes marked degrees of bone marrow hypoplasia. These patients are treated in the clinic as outpatients, and serious complications of therapy are uncommon. On the other hand, the more intensive chemotherapy of acute leukaemia and less sensitive forms of malignant disease is usually associated with severe bone marrow depression. Treatment for this is supportive because there is no known way of reversing bone marrow aplasia or of hastening its recovery. The morbidity is due mainly to infection and there is a need to be alert to the danger from the so-called opportunistic organisms. The leucopenic, immunosuppressed patient is susceptible not only to common bacterial infections but to relatively non-pathogenic organisms. As well as bacterial, there may be fungal or yeast infections, especially monilia with less often torulosis complicating the course. Viral infections with herpes simplex or herpes zoster may be severe. Respiratory infection with the protozoan *Pneumocystis carinii* is another unusual infection encountered. Gram-negative septicaemia and other life threatening infective complications are common and are frequent causes of death. Death from haemorrhage is less common. Well organised nursing care, appropriate antibiotics, blood and platelet transfusions, and sometimes granulocyte transfusions, are the basis of the supportive measures. Expert care is essential (O'Loughlin, 1975; Schimpff, 1977).

Cytotoxic agents share many other toxic side effects (Cridland, 1972). They also have a number of curiously selective adverse effects, peculiar to one drug or another, often occurring at comparable therapeutic dose levels. The common adverse effects and complications associated with cancer chemotherapy are summarised in table III.

The adverse effects are not confined to those listed. Neuropathy or stomatitis, for instance, may be caused by the nitrosoureas, but they are not a predominant feature of these drugs, whereas with methotrexate, soreness of the mouth is a common early toxic manifestation. Drug induced stomatitis is a distressing symptom for the patient especially, as may occur in acute leukaemia, when it is added to a variety of lesions of the lips and mouth related to the disease itself.

Some degree of hair loss may occur with any cytotoxic drug but it is marked, and often total, after vincristine and with higher doses of cyclophosphamide. Some adverse reactions occur only in isolated cases, such as the itchy rash that occasionally develops after procarbazine.

Treatment with cytotoxic drugs is often unpleasant for the patient although patients differ in their tolerance of the side effects and tolerance can differ from one course to the next. During the more vigorous courses of chemotherapy some patients become convinced they are more likely to die from the treatment than from the disease. Nausea and vomiting are dreaded most, especially when these symptoms persist for several days after every course of chemotherapy. Anti-emetic drugs should be given routinely to reduce the intensity of drug induced symptoms.

With vincristine temporary loss of hair seems to worry patients less than the associated neuropathy. Patients complain particularly of the numbness in their fingers. Clumsiness and weakness may also occur later. The neuropathy is usually largely reversible but can leave residual disability in older patients, and vincristine should be suspended if this toxic effect is pronounced. Vincristine can be given again after recovery, but with added caution. Symptoms tend to be less troublesome if the dose injected each time is no more than 2mg.

The cystitis from cyclophosphamide may be minimal, with a little frequency and dysuria, or haemorrhagic and lead to fibrosis of the bladder. Chlorambucil or melphalan should be substituted for cyclophosphamide if marked symptoms of cystitis develop.

Damage to the gonads may be slight or cause permanent sterility. Patients should be warned about the possible mutagenic effects upon the ovary or testis and advised against parenthood. Damage to the developing embryo is a potential hazard and if possible, cytotoxic drugs should be witheld during pregnancy, at least during the first few months. The results of cytotoxic drug therapy on the embryo are not consistent. Multiple gross fetal abnormalities may result in one case with an apparently normal infant delivered in another. The incidence of malformation is not high (Cohlan, 1969; Hemsworth and Jackson, 1965).

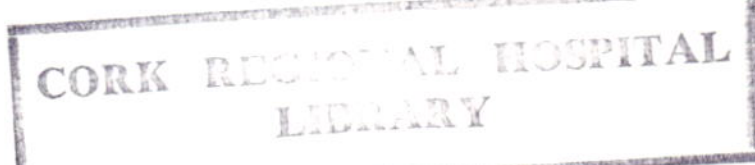

Table III. Complications of cancer chemotherapy

Adverse effect	Drugs	Comment
Damage to haemopoietic tissue	All except asparaginase	Infective and haemorrhagic complications can be fatal
Nausea and vomiting	Most	
Alopecia	Actinomycin D Adriamycin Cyclophosphamide Daunorubicin Vincristine	Some hair loss may occur with all cytotoxic drugs; reversible
Neuropathy (axonal degeneration)	Vincristine Vinblastine	Marked with vincristine; reversible; worse in elderly
Damage to mucous membranes	Actinomycin D Adriamycin Cytarabine Daunorubicin Fluorouracil Methotrexate Mitomycin	Early toxic sign with methotrexate
Cardiotoxicity	Adriamycin Daunorubicin	Cumulative, dose related
Cystitis	Cyclophosphamide	
Skin reactions	Actinomycin D Bleomycin Busulphan Hydroxyurea Mithramycin Procarbazine	Dose related pigmentation with busulphan; may be associated with a wasting syndrome; various skin lesions with other drugs
Liver dysfunction	Asparaginase Mercaptopurine Methotrexate Thioguanine	Reversible
Pneumonitis or pulmonary fibrosis	Bleomycin Busulphan Methotrexate	Reversible
Sterility and gonadal damage	Probably all cytotoxic drugs	Possibility of mutagenic effects (if not sterile); sterility may be reversible
Embryonic malformation	Probably all	Inconsistent effects
Induced malignant disease	Probably all	Long term immunosuppression in renal transplant recipients; carcinogenic in animals

Destruction of malignant cells by drug or radiation therapy causes a rise in the serum uric acid concentration which may lead to obstruction of the renal tubules and acute renal failure. Allopurinol should be given routinely when a large tumour mass is undergoing resolution. Allopurinol inhibits the degradation of mercaptopurine and the dose of the latter should be reduced when the 2 drugs are given concurrently.

Since the induction of long remissions and cure by chemotherapy have become more common, there has been renewed concern over the possibility of drug induced tumours or leukaemia. As previously mentioned, in man the danger of direct carcinogenic effects of cytotoxic drugs appears to be slight. Whatever the underlying mechanisms are, the risk of the immunosuppressed patient developing a second malignant disease is greater than would otherwise be expected, but it is not yet known whether a single course of therapy such as MOPP (see appendix) increases that risk. Acute leukaemia is the most frequent malignant condition reported to occur among patients who have had cancer chemotherapy (Reimer et al., 1977). There is of course, a natural incidence of acute leukaemia in Hodgkin's disease, lymphoma and other conditions, and the longer survival of these patients is likely to be associated with an increase in this incidence. The benefits of treatment, however, greatly outweigh the risks. In cases of malignant disease, in which chemotherapy is indicated, the chances of recurrence far exceed the likelihood of a second tumour or leukaemia. When cure has almost certainly been achieved by surgery and radiotherapy, chemotherapy may not be worth the risks (Leading Article, 1976).

Conclusions

Bone marrow depression is the greatest single hazard of cytotoxic drug therapy. Other common side effects include nausea, vomiting and alopecia. The gonads, the developing embryo and gastrointestinal epithelium are also vulnerable targets. Immunosuppression and its consequences is another serious hazard.

Chapter VI

Choice of Drug, Dose and Dose Schedule

1. Choice of Drug

The choice of drug, or drugs in a particular combination, rests primarily on clinical effectiveness and is essentially empirical. It is not known, for example, why the alkylating agents should be the most effective against ovarian carcinoma but of less value in acute leukaemia.

The choice of drug may be determined by the dose or dose schedule required. High dosage usually has an emetic effect, hence a parenteral preparation would be the drug of preference when high doses are indicated. Long term low dosage, as given in the chronic leukaemias, calls for an oral preparation.

Preference for one drug rather than a similar one is sometimes established by well conducted clinical trials. In this way melphalan became the drug of choice in the treatment of myelomatosis. Melphalan was accepted by many as the drug of choice but it is generally recognised that chlorambucil or cyclophosphamide are equally good.

Early trials established busulphan as the drug of choice at the time in the treatment of chronic myelocytic leukaemia (Haddow & Timmis, 1953). The drug seems to have a preferential effect on platelets and perhaps on immature granulocytes (Galton, 1953; Galton et al., 1958). One clinical trial comparing it with cyclophosphamide showed busulphan to be better in all respects in the management of chronic myelocytic leukaemia (Kaung et al., 1971). Another alkylating agent, mitobronitol (dibromomannitol) nevertheless compares favourably with busulphan.

Serious undesirable side effects are determining factors in the choice of a drug. The neuropathy caused by vincristine limits its use, especially in the older patient. This is an unfortunate complication of a valuable drug for which there is no ideal substitute. Vinblastine is similar and can be used instead, although it too has some neurotoxicity and is more myelotoxic than vincristine. Daunorubicin and adriamycin affect the heart and the total cardiotoxic dose of these drugs must not be exceeded (Lenaz and Page, 1976).

The thioprine, azathioprine, is converted to mercaptopurine *in vivo*. Whether justified or not, azathioprine is usually prescribed as an immunosuppressive agent while the cytotoxic antimetabolite, mercaptopurine, remains the thioprine of choice in acute leukaemia.

The choice of drug is also influenced by the prescriber's familiarity with a particular drug. One might be more familiar with the optimal dose range of melphalan in multiple myeloma while another might prefer chlorambucil or cyclophosphamide.

The choice of drugs in combination therapy also rests primarily with their clinical effectiveness as single agents. As discussed elsewhere (see chapter 7, section 2), each drug in the combination should have a different mode of action and differing side effects.

In vitro sensitivity tests with tissue cultures from the tumour have been used for many years in an attempt to aid selection of the most suitable agent. Good correlation with clinical observation is claimed. For example, in ovarian carcinoma about 50% of cell cultures show marked sensitivity to alkylating agents, which correlates well with the 50% response rate seen clinically. As might be expected, however, discrepancies occur between *in vitro* results and clinical responses. If a tumour is responding well, a conflicting sensitivity test is not a firm indication to change the treatment. Another factor may cause discrepancies: cells are grown from the tumour removed at the initial operation; the tumour may then be irradiated, and later, chemotherapy given for residual tumour or recurrence. It is quite possible that the residual or recurrent tumour has a different cell population and that the original results of sensitivity tests no longer apply.

2. Dose of Drug

In general, cell survival decreases exponentially with increasing doses, so that a suitable drug should be more effective when given in maximally tolerated dosage.

In addition to sensitivity related to the cell cycle, there is a range of inherent sensitivity. Clinically, tumours differ greatly in their response to a given dose of an effective drug, as well as having a range of sensitivity within the one tumour type. Chronic lymphocytic leukaemia may be extremely sensitive to chlorambucil, as little as 2mg daily causing a satisfactory fall in the lymphocyte count and regression of enlarged nodes and spleen. Hodgkin's disease would require 10 times that daily dose, while even larger doses would have minimal effect on most bronchogenic carcinomas.

Minimum lethal doses of drugs can be stated only approximately. It depends on the type of drug, the dose schedule and the state of the bone marrow. There is a dose range which should not be exceeded in a given single short course of treatment. A single injection of vincristine, for instance, is less likely to cause early troublesome neuropathy if the dose does not exceed 2mg. The recommended dose of mustine given alone, is 0.4mg/kg with an estimated fatal dose level of 1mg/kg.

Few of the cytotoxic drugs have definite dose related cumulative effects such as the cardiotoxicity of daunorubicin and adriamycin (Lenaz and Page, 1976). When chemotherapy was first introduced, concern was expressed about the total dose of a cytotoxic agent that could be given over a period of time. Patients with chronic lymphocytic leukaemia, for example, receiving courses of chlorambucil at a dose of 4mg daily might take a total dose of about 5g in 5 years. While long continued intake of a drug can certainly lead to irreversible bone marrow damage, the lethal dose cannot be expressed in terms of a specific total dose not to be exceeded.

A discussion of dosage cannot be dissociated from the dose schedule. Given as a single dose, a drug can cause death whereas the same dose over several weeks might have no measurable toxicity. Long term moderate daily doses have a more deleterious effect on the marrow than the same total amount given in divided doses allowing for recovery of the marrow between courses. On the other hand, a large single dose of a phase-specific drug can be far less myelotoxic than the same amount given in divided doses to affect several phases of the cell cycle. Clearly, the effect depends on the type of drug and the dose schedule. The condition of the bone marrow is another factor of importance because a safe dose for one patient can be fatal in another with impaired bone marrow function.

Equivalent dosages of various drugs are difficult to estimate accurately, even in the case of similar alkylating agents. Differences in absorption, distribution, metabolism and reactivity at a molecular level might considerably alter the actual dose delivered to the target cells.

3. Choice of Dose Schedule

The choice of dose schedule is partly empirical though based on a planned successive reduction of the malignant cell population by repeated courses of treatment. As a general principle, the higher the dose the greater the cell kill, and single high doses are more effective than long term low dose therapy. The limits of safety and undesirable side effects impose restrictions on the design and choice of all dose schedules.

Timing of the dose can be critical in the optimal control of a disease. High dosage at close intervals is the most effective way of inducing remission in acute leukaemia. A series of high dose intermittent courses of chemotherapy is optimal in Hodgkin's disease. In well differentiated lymphoma there may be a wider range of choice of effective dose schedules.

There are a few exceptions or contraindications to the use of high doses, related primarily to the state of the bone marrow. The chronic leukaemias come into this category, for on the whole, high doses of cytotoxic drugs are not well tolerated in these cases. In chronic lymphocytic leukaemia, thrombocytopenia is one of the immediate hazards in the use of high doses of alkylating agents, while drug induced neutropenia can be an added problem. Fortunately, relatively low dose courses of chlorambucil are often most effective and there is no therapeutic advantage in risking high dosage. The duration of each course depends on the response to treatment. Chlorambucil given for 2 or 3 weeks every few months may suffice, while in others, courses of a few weeks' duration may be more satisfactory. There is less tendency in recent years to prescribe low dose continuous chlorambucil, possible immunosuppression being one of the risks. The incidence of infection, however, was no greater in those patients previously treated in this way (Cridland, 1974; Galton 1959; Silver, 1969).

High dose chemotherapy is also hazardous in chronic myelocytic leukaemia. Prolonging a course of busulphan in an attempt to induce a complete bone marrow remission is also contraindicated. There have been a few reports of very long remissions after busulphan overdosage, but the outcome of such treatment is more often prolonged aplasia which can be fatal (Galton, 1969).

There are not many indications for low dose chemotherapy. In the first place, there are very few malignant diseases sensitive enough to be suppressed by low doses. Prolonged courses expose succeeding generations of sensitive normal cells, including the slowly proliferating, to the effects of cytotoxic drugs. Small lymphocytes in the G_0 state, if stimulated into antibody production would be among those affected, with resultant immunosuppression.

The interval between intensive courses of chemotherapy is determined by the recovery rate of the bone marrow, and treatment should be withheld while the marrow is actively regenerating. Meanwhile it is hoped that the tumour cells are not recovering at the same rate or faster. In several diseases it is possible to design a schedule which preserves enough bone marrow for recovery but reduces the malignant cell population selectively, and thereby induces a worthwhile remission. This has already been demonstrated quite consistently in acute lymphoblastic leukaemia of childhood and in Hodgkin's disease and with frequent cures in gestational choriocarcinoma and Burkitt's lymphoma.

The more intensive dose schedules cannot be continued safely for long periods. Six cycles of MOPP, though safe, impose a strain on the bone marrow, and cycles at intervals of 2 weeks could not be repeated indefinitely. When there are indications for continuing intensive courses of therapy for long periods, such as 18 months, 2 years or until relapse, whenever that might be, a somewhat arbitrary interval of 4 to 6 weeks is commonly chosen. Again, bone marrow toxicity is the major immediate concern and the governing factor in the planning of such schedules.

When treatment is likely to be prophylactic in a proportion of cases, it is given for the period during which the majority of recurrences can be expected. Stage II ovarian carcinoma, possibly cured by surgery, may be treated on this basis for about

2 years. In the case of possible cure in carcinoma of the breast, the patient remains at risk for very much longer. However, few clinicians favour continuing prophylactic treatment indefinitely in such cases. The patient is usually treated for only 2 years, in the hope that some 20 courses of chemotherapy might eradicate microscopic disease. In view of the immediate and possible latent complications (Leading Article, 1977; Reimer et al., 1977) prophylactic chemotherapy may not be justified unless the risk of recurrence is high.

There is no unanimity in the design of maintenance therapy, if any, during long remissions of diseases in which cure is not anticipated. Lymphocytic lymphoma can remain apparently dormant for years. It may be argued that some form of regular maintenance chemotherapy might keep it dormant for longer. The opposite view holds that treatment is unnecessary, or could even do harm, when natural host defences appear to be in some control of the disease.

Slight adjustment of dose levels which are already of a low order is safe and common practice in the management of the chronic leukaemias and related disorders. There are a few other dose schedules in which progressively increasing doses are advocated, but in general, increasing the dose of a cytotoxic drug during a course of treatment is not recommended. A marrow already depressed by treatment does not easily withstand a sudden increase in dosage unless, of course, that increase is very small.

In clinical trials to compare the effectiveness of different drugs, the dose schedule alone can be critical. Dose schedules should therefore be similar if valid comparisons are to be made between one drug and another.

4. Conclusions

The choice of drug depends primarily on the sensitivity of the tumour and is largely empirical. The choice is also influenced by dose requirements, dose schedules and most suitable combinations.

In general, the higher the dose, the greater the cell kill, and high dose intermittent chemotherapy is the dose schedule of choice in most cases. Toxicity of the drugs is the limiting factor in the design of dose schedules.

Chapter VII

Single Drug and Combination Chemotherapy

1. Single Drug Treatment

Two drugs are not necessarily better than one. Single drugs are used alone when a disease is sensitive to only one agent or its derivatives, with little or no clinical sensitivity to other types of drug. They are also used alone when no advantage with multiple drug therapy can be demonstrated.

Choriocarcinoma and Burkitt's lymphoma are both curable by single drug therapy, although both these tumours respond well to several different agents. Single drugs, such as mercaptopurine and methotrexate, also have a place in the maintenance therapy of acute leukaemia.

Chronic lymphocytic leukaemia is usually very sensitive to quite small doses of alkylating agents. Chlorambucil alone is very effective and there seems to be no therapeutic gain in combining it with vincristine. If response is poor and dose requirements for chlorambucil approach toxic levels, the combination is worth trying, but the results are usually disappointing.

Lymphocytic lymphoma also responds better to alkylating agents than to other types of cytotoxic drug and excellent results are attainable with courses of chlorambucil or cyclophosphamide alone. Certainly in some cases of lymphocytic lymphoma the combination of alkylating agent and prednisone is better. The more malignant lymphomas are better controlled by combination therapy and this may eventually prove to be so in the well differentiated forms. When vincristine causes marked neuropathy, as sometimes occurs in the elderly, its use is contraindicated. Side effects from prednisone may preclude its use also. Under these conditions an alkylating agent alone can be given with good effect.

Combination therapy has perhaps not yet been given a fair trial in ovarian carcinoma, but so far it appears that alkylating agents alone are the most effective, with a remission rate of 50%. The antimetabolite fluorouracil causes regression in 25 to 30% of cases while other types of agent have a success range of 5 to 15%. Some advantage might be expected to accrue from the combined use of several agents, and further trials may clarify the place of combination chemotherapy in ovarian carcinoma.

In comparing the relative value of single drugs with combination chemotherapy, variables should be reduced to a minimum. Similar dose schedules should be used for valid comparisons. It is meaningless to compare the effect of a single course of a single drug with the effect of several drugs given in a series of courses and to conclude that the single drug is inferior. Several courses of that single drug might have an effect equal to the combination and should be tried in the same way before being dismissed as inferior treatment. There are usually, however, greater limits on dosage when single drugs are used.

2. Combination Chemotherapy

Combination chemotherapy refers to the concurrent, and to some extent sequential, use of several drugs in an attempt to achieve maximum therapeutic effect without increasing unduly the undesirable side effects (Carter and Soper, 1974; De Vita and Schein, 1973).

There are a large number of combinations known by bewildering abbreviations such as MOPP, MVPP, COPP, COP, CVP, VAMP, TRIKE, CMF, COMB, CHOP and others, plus many more to come. Vincristine provides the vowel 'O' because of its proprietary name 'Oncovin.' The letter C usually represents cyclophosphamide, while M can mean mustine, methotrexate, mercaptopurine, methyl-CCNU (semustine) or any other drug beginning with 'M'. Some of the more frequently used combinations of drugs are listed in the appendix.

Drug combinations should fulfill certain criteria:

1) Each drug in the combination should be active when used alone against the tumour
2) The drugs should have different modes of action
3) The toxic side effects should differ

For example, lymphocytic lymphoma is sensitive to alkylating agents, vincristine and prednisone, and each of these drugs has a different mode of action and different effect on the cell cycle. The therapeutic dose of vincristine is less myelotoxic than a comparable dose of an alkylating agent but vincristine is neurotoxic. By combining the two it is possible to deliver a more effective and higher therapeutic dose without a proportional increase in toxicity to normal cells. Prednisone is lymphocytolytic and does not impair bone marrow function. The trio makes up the combination COP (Bonadonna and Monfardini, 1974; Ultmann, 1970; Ultmann and Nixon, 1969).

Combination therapy has particular relevance in Hodgkin's disease, one best treated by high dose intermittent chemotherapy. The use of MOPP (mustine, 'Oncovin' [vincristine], procarbazine and prednisone) has proved to be most effective. The cycle-specific alkylating agents are the basis of treatment of Hodgkin's disease. It also responds well to procarbazine which behaves rather like an alkylating agent. The phase-specific vinca alkaloids are also active against Hodgkin's disease (De Vita et al., 1970; De Vita et al., 1972; Rubens et al., 1972). The value of prednisone is debatable for it offers only transient benefit, if any, when used alone. Some clinical observations have suggested that MOPP is superior to MOP (without the prednisone) [Jeliffe, 1975]. Prednisone has been shown to enhance the effect of vincristine in some experimental systems, but the need for prednisone in MOPP for Hodgkin's disease has not yet been established.

The success of combination therapy owes much to the dose schedules employed. MOPP delivers a succession of high dose, short term cycles of chemotherapy at 2 week intervals, which are usually adequate to permit bone marrow recovery between each cycle and at the same time deal effectively with the disease. In acute myeloblastic leukaemia, 7 days of cytarabine with daunorubicin on days 1, 2 and 3, repeated a week or so later on a 5 and 2 day schedule is often adequate to induce a remission. The margin of safety is narrow but the treatment is selective enough to preserve sufficient normal marrow for recovery and at the same time induce a good remission in some 50% of cases.

The presumed presence of resistant or less sensitive cell lines in a given malignant cell population is another reason offered for using combination chemotherapy. Two or more drugs usually have a wider spectrum of activity than one drug alone. There is always the chance that some of the less sensitive cells can be suppressed or at least have their emergence delayed.

This raises the argument of using all kinds of drugs in combination without particular regard to the apparent sensitivity of the tumour at the time. There has been some controversy in the medical literature over the inclusion of clinically ineffective cytotoxic drugs in combination chemotherapy (Bunn, 1974). Examples have been quoted of single drugs being of no value alone but successful when combined with another effective drug. It is possible that one drug might alter the conditions so that another is able to exert its cytotoxic effect, but it is difficult to assess the contribution of each drug. With such a combination, added unwanted toxicity is a certainty while the conferring of therapeutic value on an otherwise ineffective drug is unlikely.

Initial therapy should always be directed against the known sensitivity of the tumour and should include only those drugs documented or demonstrated to be active when used alone. In practice, the resistant cells that do ultimately emerge in the course of a disease are only too frequently resistant to all chemotherapeutic agents.

The terms additive and synergistic should be applied with caution, especially in the clinical sense. These effects are also subject to different interpretations. They may be defined in biochemical terms or by the survival of cells in suspension exposed to cytotoxic drugs, or by the lifespan of animals or patients. It is very difficult, even in the experimental system, to assay the contribution made by each drug in a combination. Clinically, there is really no way of assessing whether the observed effects are additive, synergistic or even due to one drug only.

Combined drug effects in the algebraic sense is the concept commonly held. If one drug kills 20% of cells and another 50% while the combination kills 70%, the result may be said to be additive. If fewer than 30% survive, the combined effect may be synergistic. The figures are meaningless if both drugs kill off 90%. The conclusions are simplistic and far from the truth: there is the effect of the dosage to consider and the dose survival curves; there is the dose schedule and the interaction between the agents used; finally there is the phase specificity of the drugs to be taken into account and the effects upon the target cells that are out of phase or out of reach in a state of G_0.

Certain drug combinations may be less than additive in their cytotoxic effects. Methotrexate can increase the intracellular deoxycytidine triphosphate pool which protects the cells from the effect of cytarabine. Methotrexate also increases the level of deoxyuridylic acid thus reducing the effectiveness of fluorouracil. These reactions were detected in cell cultures, and the observed results might not apply in the whole animal (Tattersall et al., 1973; Tattersall et al., 1974; Tattersall and Harrap, 1973). In other studies with L1210 leukaemia cells, enhanced cytotoxicity was observed with the combination of methotrexate and fluorouracil, probably due to the sequential blockade of thymidylate synthetase to produce a marked reduction in DNA synthesis (Goldin, 1971). In clinical practice, the choice of effective drugs in combination is still largely empirical, but the clinician should be aware of disadvantageous possibilities when designing combined chemotherapy regimens. If two useful drugs are likely to be antagonistic, they might best be given sequentially. As discussed in chapter III, many factors influence the biological effects of the various drugs on the target cells.

The number of effective drugs in a combination is usually no more than 4, but up to 8 are included in a few of the better known regimens. As the number is increased, modifications in dosage are needed to avoid an excessive total dose. Whereas in experimental systems the optimal dose range of each drug can be demonstrated and the efficacy of multiple drug combinations more readily assessed, this is not so clinically. In clinical studies undertaken by Acute Leukaemia Group B, 3-drug regimens compared unfavourably with 4-drug regimens in the treatment of Hodgkin's disease. It was also noted however, that the latter were more toxic. It cannot be assumed that a combination of 3 effective drugs is necessarily inferior to a combination of 4 or 5. As part of the same study, MOPP was compared with a 5-drug combination of chlorambucil, vincristine, vinblastine, procarbazine and prednisone and with a 4-drug combination in which mustine was replaced by chlorambucil. The dose schedule was similar in the 3 regimens, and the overall response rate was close to 90% in all 3 routines (Nissen et al., 1973). Bunn et al. (1977) found that their results of chemotherapy in small cell bronchogenic carcinoma were best with a 3- or 4-drug combination, and not improved by the use of more than 4 drugs.

While some undesirable side effects can be reduced by combining different drugs at appropriate dose levels, it should not be inferred that combination chemotherapy is without serious toxicity. There may be less chance of irreversible bone marrow depression occurring when agents of different classes are employed, but the margin of safety is often narrow. No form of cancer chemotherapy is completely safe.

Chapter VIII

Routes of Administration

1. Oral and Intravenous Administration

Most cytotoxic drugs are given intravenously or by mouth. A few, such as bleomycin, can be injected intramuscularly or, as with cytarabine, subcutaneously.

The oral route is convenient but unsuitable when high, emetic doses are required. Also, if there is any doubt about the patient's reliability in taking medication, the intravenous route is the better method of administration.

Many of the intravenous preparations can cause a severe local inflammatory reaction if they leak from the vein into the tissues. Pain and swelling can persist at the site for a couple of weeks, and the vein itself become sclerosed.

2. Intracavity Administration

Alkylating agents such as mustine or thiotepa can be given directly into the thoracic or abdominal cavity. It is still quite common practice to use thiotepa for extensive involvement of the peritoneum with ovarian carcinoma at the time of operation. Mustine is occasionally given for recurrent pleural effusion in cases of lymphoma.

Intracavity administration of alkylating agents may offer no advantage over the intravenous or oral route. There may also be the problem of lack of uniform distribution of the drug in the presence of adhesions, localised collections of fluid and tumour masses. The effect on the marrow depends upon how much of the drug is fixed or inactivated locally, and how much is absorbed and redistributed; under either circumstance it can be therapeutically active.

Intrathecal administration, usually of methotrexate, is used for meningeal involvement in acute leukaemia. Cytarabine also, is occasionally given in this way.

3. Infusions and Perfusions

The perfusion technique is a method by which cytotoxic drugs can be delivered, in relatively high concentration, to one region of the body such as a limb. The area is isolated using extracorporeal circulation so that the rest of the body is protected from the effects of the drug.

Infusion through the arterial supply of the affected part is another way in which a high local concentration of a drug can be obtained. This latter procedure is less time consuming and does not require extracorporeal circulation. A refinement of this method involves the systemic administration of the specific antidote to the drug used for infusion, as in the use of methotrexate with folinic acid (citrovorum or leucovorum factor). Some degree of bone marrow depression occurs, even with the addition of folinic acid.

Infusions may be given as a single dose or long term over a few days. Methotrexate, fluorouracil and alkylating agents are the drugs most commonly used. Tumours of the head and neck, especially recurrent squamous cell carcinoma of the tongue and floor of the mouth, have made up the majority of cases in large series treated in this way. Local reaction is usual, with varying degrees of oedema and necrosis, and tracheostomy may be needed. Temporary but worthwhile palliation can be obtained and pain relief is one of the outstanding benefits. Hepatic artery infusion for advanced metastatic disease of the liver or for hepatoma has met with some success, and infusion for melanoma localised to limbs has produced some good results (Irvine and Luck, 1966; Oberfield, 1975; Stewart, 1970).

4. Chemotherapy by Topical Application

Solutions of mustine can penetrate the skin to a depth of 1 cm and are occasionally used in mycosis fungoides and lymphomatous skin infiltrations.

Selected cases of basal cell carcinoma, Bowen's disease of the skin, leukoplakia on lips and vulva and extensive solar keratoses can be treated with topical fluorouracil. A 5% ointment is applied daily for a month or less, depending on the site and extent of the lesions. Quite severe local inflammatory reaction can result and the treatment should only be undertaken by dermatologists experienced in its use (Anderson et al., 1969; Belisario, 1969).

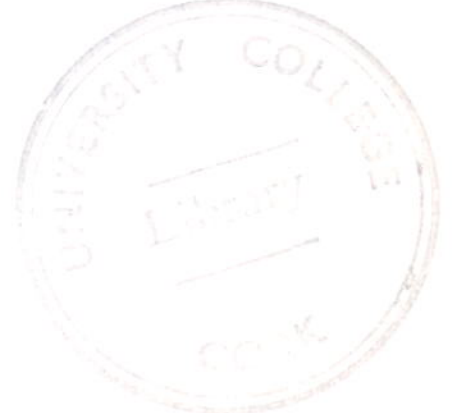

Chapter IX

The Natural History of Malignant Disease and its Response to Treatment

1. The Natural History of Malignant Disease

An appreciation of the natural history of a disease is essential in planning treatment and in assessing the results. The effect of treatment can be more readily evaluated in diseases that tend to be uniform and predictable in their behaviour. Long remissions and long survival are exceptional in acute myeloblastic leukaemia, for example, and the benefits from future satisfactory methods will be readily recognised. Results of treatment are more difficult to interpret in carcinoma of the breast, for not only is the disease more variable, but staging at diagnosis may be inaccurate.

Even in the more predictable conditions there are exceptional cases. Unexpected good results may be due more to the unusual nature of the disease in a particular case than to the treatment given. Unknown factors within the patient's immunological capabilities may augment therapy. Success might also be due to fortuitous timing of treatment. Before claims can be made for the value or superiority of a form of treatment the results must be reproducible and reviewed in relation to the natural history of the disease.

2. Response to Treatment

In comparing the relative value of chemotherapy in various disorders, the term 'response' should be defined with respect to its extent and duration and the subsequent course of the disease. A complete remission in acute leukaemia may last only a few weeks and the patient die after the first relapse. The symptomatic patient with chronic lymphocytic leukaemia on the other hand, may have only a partial haematological remission but remain fit and well for many years.

Response is sometimes described as a percentage decrease in the size of measurable tumours. If a 50% reduction were to occur in a new case of Hodgkin's disease, the result would be scored as poor. If the patient had a melanoma or renal carcinoma, a 50% reduction in the size of metastases would be a most encouraging result for chemotherapy.

Subjective improvement alone is a much less reliable measure of response to treatment. It is often most difficult to assess unless it is striking or accompanied by some objective evidence of improvement, or at least perhaps, no evidence of continuing deterioration. While there are a few patients who will never admit to feeling well in spite of complete remissions, there are many who try to feel better in spite of no demonstrable benefit from treatment.

Chapter X

Clinical Trials

The clinical value of new drugs and new regimens is assessed by clinical trial. These are difficult to design and the results may be difficult to interpret. It is important to appreciate the purpose of a trial, and its limitations, and it may take years of reapeated testing to prove which is the best therapeutic method (Hill, 1967).

Clinical trials are often cooperative studies at different centres, requiring general unanimity of the participants. While it is necessary to keep to the protocol laid down, some provision must be made to modify therapy when it is in the best interests of the patient.

The patient should be given the option of being in a clinical trial. Some are eager to try new forms of treatment whereas others refuse to be 'guinea pigs' and their feelings must be respected. In controlled trials it should be explained to the patient that his allocation to one treatment or another is not known to be disadvantageous, otherise there would be no point in conducting a trial.

When a new drug is being tested for its spectrum of activity it is common practice to include mainly patients with advanced malignant disease. These initial series include perhaps several cases of bronchogenic carcinoma, lymphomas, two or three cases of carcinoma of the colon, breast or pancreas, and a few rare tumours. The diseases are usually beyond the scope of known forms of chemotherapy and response to the new drug is a significant result worth pursuing further. Clearly these studies are only preliminary clinical screening tests and it cannot be concluded that the drug under trial is without value if no response is noted. New drugs or new regimens need to undergo extensive trials which include patients with less advanced disease, and those who have not previously been treated with chemotherapy.

When clinical trials of new drugs have been done to test their efficacy against a variety of malignant diseases, further trials may then be needed to establish the right dose schedule for those diseases that respond well. Unless a new drug is obviously much better than those already in current use, trials to compare its relative value need to be undertaken. The new drug may also be a useful addition to multiple drug regimens and further trials have to be done to test it in this regard. Meanwhile, of course, its value in the less sensitive diseases should be re-assessed using different schedules or combinations.

Retrospective comparisons may not be valid and appropriate contemporaneous control series are usually required. In comparing results of one trial with another or with a control series, variables in the method can confuse the issue. For example, the use of melphalan in breast cancer has been unfavourably compared with the use of 3 or 4 drugs in combination, the conclusion being that combined therapy is superior to an alkylating agent alone. The conclusion is almost certainly correct. However, comparison was made between a 5-day course of oral melphalan given every 6 weeks and intravenous triple or quadruple therapy given every 3 weeks. The dose and dose schedule themselves could be the important factors (Bonadonna et al., 1976; Broder and Carbone, 1970; Fisher, 1977; Fisher et al., 1975).

When comparing different types of treatment, case selection is an important variable that can influence results. It should be noted, for instance, whether a series of patients treated for acute leukaemia includes the very old or the very young. Different histopathological classification within a group of cases is another variable that may invalidate comparisons. In more recent years with better staging of Hodgkin's disease, patients with early stage III are treated with chemotherapy whereas formerly only those with advanced disease were referred for treatment.

When a therapeutic method is to be fully assessed, the patient should receive adequate treatment and this might take weeks or months to complete. Patients who do not live long enough to receive the prescribed minimum are necessarily withdrawn from the trial. Such selection is an acceptable procedure but it would be pointless to compare the results with those from a series which was not selected in this way and included patients with the worst prognosis.

Chapter XI

Sensitivity and Resistance to Cytotoxic Drugs

Resistance to cytotoxic drugs may be natural to the tumour or develop during the course of the disease. Natural resistance is common, in fact many of the common tumours respond poorly. Even in diseases notably sensitive to chemotherapy there are always cases which fail to respond well.

The drugs also have selectivity towards normal tissues some, such as bone marrow cells, being highly sensitive to most cytotoxic drugs. It is unknown why drugs that can disrupt DNA or inhibit its synthesis should be so selective. Biochemical differences in the target cells is thought to be one of the most likely explanations.

Most studies on sensitivity and resistance to cytotoxic drugs and their selectivity have been done on the effects of antimetabolites on isolated cell systems or other experimental models, and there is little information about these mechanisms in tumours in humans. No doubt the same mechanisms operate, but the system is much more complex in the clinical situation (Bender and Dedrick, 1975; Hill and Baserga, 1975).

Among the many factors that could affect a tumour's response to chemotherapeutic agents are included the size and site of the tumour and its blood supply. The dose, dose schedule and route of administration of the drugs also influence access to the tumour and its response.

At a cellular level, the nature of the cell membrane can affect uptake, transport and retention of a drug. Inactivation of drugs by enzyme systems, changes in the enzyme systems themselves and competitive removal of a drug by reaction with other molecules are possible ways in which sensitivity to treatment might be modified (Ball, 1969). In the case of methotrexate, for instance, resistance is due to at least two of these mechanisms (Harrap et al., 1971). Impaired transport of methotrexate and increase in the total dihydrofolate reductase level have been demonstrated in mammalian cell cultures. The effects of the mixed cell population in the environment is another complex factor that could influence the cytotoxicity of a drug towards target cells, and which cannot readily be demonstrated *in vitro*. Induced mutagenic changes have also been suggested as a possible mechanism which could change the sensitivity to a drug.

Inhibition of *de novo* synthesis of DNA by antimetabolites may initiate utilisation of alternate metabolic pathways, with incorporation of preformed nucleosides and bases. The outcome would be influenced by the relative dependence of tissues on *de novo* or salvage pathways and the availability of appropriate metabolites for DNA biosynthesis.

Less is known about the factors determining sensitivity and resistance to alkylating agents. It has been demonstrated in bacteria, and some other experimental systems, that damage to DNA can be repaired by processes called excision repair and post-replication repair. Whether clinical failure of response is due to resistance acquired by these mechanisms is largely unknown.

Resistance must also be viewed within the context of the natural history of the disease and the heterogenicity of most malignant cell populations. Less sensitive cells can be selected out by treatment so that the tumour becomes a predominantly resistant population of cells. Skipper (1974) demonstrated that a leukaemic cell population surviving exposure to cytarabine was in fact resistant to that drug. The use of appropriate combination therapy with several drugs should lessen the chance of emergence of resistant populations of cells because two drugs can have a greater range of activity than one.

Acquired resistance need not be drug induced because in the course of their natural history, many tumours become progressively less differentiated and less responsive, irrespective of previous treatment. The use of busulphan in chronic myelocytic leukaemia does not seem to hasten the development of blastic transformation. The change is part of the natural history of the disease and occurs whether the patient is treated or not.

There appears to be no justification for the practice of withholding drugs in case they induce early resistance. If true drug induced resistance can occur, it is difficult to demonstrate it as the cause of failed response. If it is likely to occur, it is not predictable. Repeated good response to the same treatment may continue for years in lymphoma, for instance. In another case of the same type, the lymphoma may change its behaviour early in its course and become rapidly progressive and resist all known forms of treatment. Whatever mechanisms are involved it is difficult to accept the concept of drug induced resistance acquired only by malignant cells while the bone marrow and other sensitive normal tissues remain eternally vulnerable.

Resistance to chemotherapy can be localised to one area. After treatment of generalised disease, all enlarged nodes may regress except one. In another case, one lymph node may rapidly enlarge again without demonstrable signs of recurrence elsewhere. Radiotherapy is usually the next treatment of choice in cases of apparently localised resistance.

Response appears to depend not only on the inherent nature of a disease but also on the patient's immune competence to cope with that disease. How interdependent all these factors might be is yet to be clarified. It is well documented that impaired immune competence can be associated with a poor prognosis and that progression of malignant disease may be accompanied by a decline in a variety of immune responses. While treatment with chemotherapy may also cause immunosuppression, a rebound phenomenon has been observed in some cases. It has also been suggested that the drugs might reduce the blocking antibody-antigen complexes that protect a tumour but the mechanism is not really known.

Not infrequently poor response is wrongly attributed to resistance when in fact it is due to inadequate dosage or suboptimal dose schedules. Relapse during maintenance therapy too, does not necessarily imply that resistance to that drug has developed. The maintenance dose might be quite inadequate and the remission due entirely to the initial course of chemotherapy. For this reason the drug need not be deleted permanently from future treatment schedules.

In the treatment of acute leukaemia there is a tendency to discard drugs that were effective before relapse on the assumption that all subsequent relapses comprise resistant cell populations. While there is a good case for putting aside those drugs for the time being while other treatment is tried, it cannot be assumed that they no longer have a place in the management of future relapses. The nature of ermerging or reemerging cell populations is not known, but it seems unlikely that previous treatment has entirely eliminated the earlier sensitive cell lines. It is worth trying some drugs again in the course of acute leukaemia.

It is nevertheless true that failure of response during a course of previously effective treatment is a poor prognostic sign in any malignant disease. Certainly a change in treatment may deal effectively with any change in the malignant process, but as a general rule the chances of complete remission ultimately become progressively less. Perhaps the disease becomes refractory partly as a result of the patient's immune response failing to augment the effect of cytotoxic drugs.

Conclusions

Resistance to cytotoxic drugs may be inherent in the tumour or develop during the course of a disease. Many factors may influence resistance or sensitivity to treatment. An important factor in the development of a resistant cell population may be the selecting out of less sensitive cells.

Chapter XII

General Management

1. Blood Counts

Blood counts and bone marrow examinations are part of the diagnostic procedure in leukaemia and most other so-called haematological disorders, and they are also done before chemotherapy is prescribed for any reason.

Treatment entails strict supervision of the patient because of the dangers associated with cytotoxic drug therapy. Fortunately changes in the peripheral blood provide a fairly reliable guide to the degree of myelosuppression caused by the drugs. Repeat bone marrow examinations may also be necessary during courses of therapy, especially in acute leukaemia.

The frequency with which blood counts are done depends on the dosage and the disease. When treatment is aggressive, or the marrow infiltrated with malignant cells, counts may be necessary every few days. In a stabilised case of chronic leukaemia, a count every 6 weeks or so is often adequate.

Any changes in the blood count resulting from treatment of relapse in leukaemia can be more readily appreciated by plotting the counts on some kind of chart. A chart based on a semilogarithmic scale, designed by Hart and recommended by Galton in 1959, is most useful in this regard (fig. 2). The rise and fall of the cell counts are exponential in character and form straight lines on charts based on this scale. Predictions can be made with reasonable accuracy by extrapolation and dosage can be adjusted accordingly.

Figure 2 is a simplified version of part of a chart of a patient with chronic myelocytic leukaemia. The white cell count fell steeply under the influence of busulphan 4mg daily, with a change in rate of fall when the dose was reduced. In this case there was an early tendency for the count to rise, with reappearance of immature granulocytes whenever the drug was suspended. Subsequently courses of busulphan

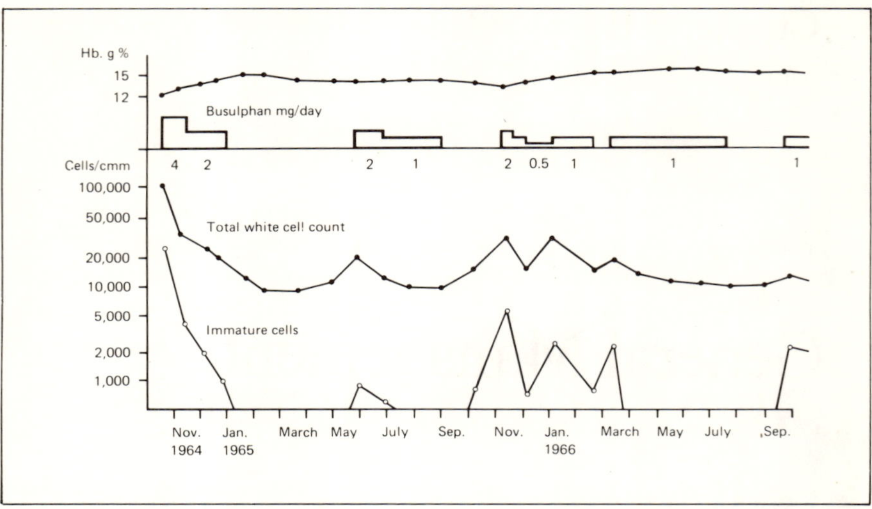

Fig. 2. Blood count chart showing the effect of busulphan and the white cells of a patient with chronic myelocytic leukaemia.

1 mg a day for 4 weeks, at intervals of about 4 weeks, proved to be adequate in keeping the blood count within normal limits. Charts of this kind are also useful as a case summary which can be assessed at a glance.

2. Instructions to the Patient Receiving Cytotoxic Drugs

All patients should be warned about the dangers of overdosage and told why regular blood counts are necessary. Better informed patients are more cooperative. Without information some non-leukaemic patients get the idea they have leukaemia as well as the disease they are being treated for.

The majority adhere to instructions but perhaps in most cases it is wiser to prescribe only the required amount of tablets for a single course of treatment, thus avoiding confusion and any risk of overdosage.

Patients should be warned about nausea and vomiting and other possible side effects such as oral ulceration from methotrexate. They should be told about alopecia and even the bald man should be forwarned about the loss of his few cherished hairs.

Patients usually like to know the outcome of discussions of their case and they should be kept informed. However, on ward rounds it is preferable to discuss each case beyond the sight and hearing of the patient. A solemn group of doctors whispering at the foot of the bed is hardly reassuring to the patient already apprehensive about his disease and its treatment; what the patient fails to hear, those in neighbouring beds will strain their ears to catch, and then relay the information in fragmented form.

Most patients want to know the diagnosis and prognosis, at least in general terms. The vast majority adapt to the situation with surprising fortitude. It is a mistake, however, to state the prognosis initially in precise numbers of weeks, months or years, because the patient will count them and the estimation of his survival could be quite inaccurate. While some patients triumphantly recall they were given 6 months to live 6 years ago, those 6 years would have been more enjoyable without knowledge of the silent reaper's presence.

3. Who Should Treat the Patient?

It is preferable that patients receiving cancer chemotherapy are managed by those experienced in the use of cytotoxic drugs. Special hospitals or special units within general hospitals are organised to administer appropriate treatment for the diseases and their complications. With the use of more intensive chemotherapy, dealing with the complications of treatment has become an increasing part of management. Facilities such as barrier nursing, the ready availability of blood, platelets and so on, and expert help from laboratory and radiology departments are essential. The management of patients with acute leukaemia illustrates the problem well, and it can be done satisfactorily only in well equipped hospitals with well trained staff. The ultimate decisions rest with the clinician in charge of the case, but the overall management involves team work.

The general practitioner, or specialist who has referred the patient, should be kept informed of the nature of the treatment given and the variety of adverse reactions that might occur. The country practitioner in particular has added responsibilities, sometimes including his direct participation in the chemotherapeutic management.

The treatment of malignant disease is the province of the surgeon, radiotherapist, clinical haematologist and oncologist, the majority of patients being treated long term by one of the three last mentioned. It is unfortunate that patients are often treated by different groups of specialists in separate clinics. Those with leukaemia, lymphoma and the myeloproliferative disorders tend to be referred to the haematology clinics, and the so-called solid tumours for chemotherapy are treated by the oncologists. The radiotherapists continue to deal with a wider range of malignant disease and have usually had considerable experience in chemotherapy. Physicians in the field of cancer chemotherapy must have some training in the radiotherapy departments to appreciate the scope of radiation therapy, not only in the treatment of localised disease but of patients with generalised disease as well. Conjoint clinics with representatives from the various specialties have obvious advantages.

4. To Treat or Not to Treat

When the possibility of benefit from chemotherapy is remote, debate may arise over the decision to treat or not to treat the patient. The problem presents itself in those cases in which cytotoxic agents so far tried are no longer effective or in those malignant diseases in which chemotherapy is known to have little value. If there is a reasonable chance of benefit from a new drug or different combination, the treatment should of course, be tried. In the event of progressive disease, in spite of attempts to control it, chemotherapy should be stopped.

It is not easy to withhold specific treatment from patients, particularly those who are fully aware of the situation. However, the desire 'to do something' is not an indication to prescribe expensive drugs that could make the patient's remaining weeks a misery. Repeated attempts to achieve a remission will only result in marrow aplasia and septicaemia which might well shorten the patient's survival.

In practice, most previously treated patients are leucopenic by the time the final stages of their illnesses are reached; this provides a legitimate reason for not giving any further chemotherapy, a reason also that the patient understands. Apathy is often associated with debilitating disease and patients tend to lose their will to live during the late stages. Some actually request no further treatment, especially the emetic combinations of drugs that make up so much of cancer chemotherapy today. Those few who ask for treatment and could withstand further chemotherapy, are sometimes admitted to clinical trials of new drugs or new methods. Appropriate clinical trials in progress might influence the decision to treat patients with diseases resistant to known methods of chemotherapy. This is not meant to imply that patients with terminal illness should be directed into the more experimental realms of medicine. It is merely a suggested alternative for the selected few, not the dying majority.

5. Terminal Care

When specific treatment is no longer of benefit, the patient must be sustained with appropriate supportive measures. These measures are designed for the patient's comfort and rarely appreciably prolong life.

How far medical aid should go in an attempt to prolong life in the dying patient is a recurring question, but there are limitations to the effectiveness of supportive measures in this regard. Relief of pain and anxiety, adequate hydration and expert nursing care are essential for the patient's comfort. If he is distressed by anaemia, a blood transfusion might be indicated, but quite often it fails to produce the desired effect.

If patients cannot be nursed at home, ideally they should be admitted to the hospital they have been attending during their illness, but beds for this purpose may not be available. Where patients are cared for at this stage depends on the nature of the illness. Most with acute leukaemia die in hospital where attempts are being made to cure septicaemia or other complications. Intestinal obstruction and other acute emergencies of malignant disease may also be reasons for admission to hospital. Many patients, however, linger on for weeks and may need more attention than their relatives can provide at home.

'Disposal of the patient', as it is called, is a term not recommended for use within earshot of the patient or his relatives. Transfer to a suitable nursing home is, however, the only way in which some patients can be given the care they need. There are many nursing homes staffed by those skilled in terminal care and although patients may be well aware of their fate, most come to terms with it and prefer the nursing home to the hospital environment.

6. Conclusions

Regular blood counts are essential during cytotoxic drug therapy, and the general principles of treatment should be explained to the patient.

Patients are best managed by units experienced in the treatment of malignant disease. The desire 'to do something' for the dying patient is not an indication for chemotherapy.

Chapter XIII

Acute Leukaemia

The approach to the treatment of acute leukaemia has changed radically from cautious palliation to aggressive drug therapy (Farber et al., 1948; Henderson, 1967; Holland, 1969). Treatment aims at the differential destruction of the leukaemic cell population, preserving enough normal haemopoietic tissue to regenerate. Vigorous supportive measures are an essential part of the treatment during the phase of severe bone marrow depression. Improved supportive measures have contributed to the better survival figures.

Having achieved remission, consolidation therapy then maintenance therapy may be given with the intention of destroying remaining abnormal cells while their numbers are reduced. Immunotherapy is added in the hope of destroying the last surviving leukaemic cells, or at least of enhancing the effect of chemotherapy (Bernard and Boiron, 1970).

The outlook has greatly improved in most cases of childhood lymphoblastic leukaemia. The median survival is now 3 years and continues to increase. The figures based on cases of long term survival suggest that of those who survive 5 years without relapse, some 50% might be cured. The outlook remains bleak in the acute myeloblastic form. In adults the prognosis is somewhat better in the less common lymphoblastic leukaemia than in the acute myeloblastic, but the overall results are most unsatisfactory (Gunz and Vincent, 1977; Henderson, 1969; Jacquillat et al., 1973; Mathe, 1970; Walters, 1976).

1. Acute Lymphoblastic Leukaemia

Prednisone and weekly injections of vincristine are used to induce remission, which is achieved in most children within 6 weeks. In the 5% or so in whom remission does not occur, daunorubicin, adriamycin or cytarabine may be added to the induction regimen.

After remission has been induced, the cranium is irradiated; intrathecal methotrexate may also be given to eradicate meningeal involvement if present in the early stages.

Consolidation therapy with further courses of vincristine and prednisone may be given for a few weeks, although the necessity for consolidation remains controversial.

Methotrexate and mercaptopurine, in repetitive cycles, are prescribed as maintenance therapy, sometimes with cyclophosphamide or vincristine. Occasional booster courses of vincristine and prednisone are advocated by some. The optimal duration of maintenance therapy is not yet known, and there is concern over possible adverse effects from long term chemotherapy (Holland and Glidewell, 1972; Mathe, 1969; Simone et al., 1972; Walters, 1976).

Immunotherapy with BCG and allogeneic cells has been used by Mathe with favourable results in acute lymphoblastic leukaemia. Others have found immunotherapy of greater potential value in acute myeloblastic leukaemia (Crowther et al., 1973; Heyn et al., 1973; MRC, 1971; Powles, 1976).

Lymphoblastic leukaemia in adults is treated similarly, but without comparably good results.

2. Acute Myeloblastic Leukaemia

The drugs used in various dose schedules include cytarabine, daunorubicin, adriamycin, thioguanine, mercaptopurine, vincristine, cyclophosphamide, prednisone and asparaginase. Carmustine (BCNU) and lomustine (CCNU) are among more recent additions to the long list.

The protocols are often known by abbreviations such as COAP (cyclophosphamide, 'Oncovin' [vincristine], ara-C [cytarabine] and prednisone). The first was VAMP (vincristine, amethopterin, mercaptopurine and prednisone) for use in childhood leukaemia. One of the most popular and effective regimens at present used combines cytarabine and daunorubicin for induction of remission and consolidation, using cytarabine and thioguanine as conveniently administered maintenance therapy. Methotrexate and mercaptopurine are also used as maintenance drugs.

There are several variations in the dose schedule. Cytarabine may be given for 7 days and daunorubicin for 3 days in the so-called 'seven-three' regimen. A further course or two, usually of shorter duration, may be given after 5 days or so as part of the induction therapy or as consolidation when remission has been induced. The complete remission rate is about 50% but remissions rarely last more than a few months (Crowther et al., 1970).

Immunotherapy can prolong remissions in some cases and there are many trials in progress to evaluate its place in the treatment of acute leukaemia and other diseases. Studies to improve methods of immunotherapy are also being undertaken (Powles, 1976).

The prognosis is worse in the older age group; especially if the patient is frail is he unlikely to tolerate the treatment and its complications and in fact in such cases radical treatment is more likely to shorten survival. Some such patients should be given a modified form of chemotherapy while others are best treated with supportive measures only.

3. Failure of Response in Acute Leukaemia

There are many patients who do not have a haematological remission and whose marrows remain infiltrated with blast cells in spite of repeated courses of chemotherapy. Failure to achieve a remission initially is not a good sign. Treatment with different drugs and different dose schedules should certainly be tried but repeated attempts require long periods in hospital with life threatening complications of therapy. To retreat to less vigorous measures is no easy decision for the optimistic therapist, but it may be in the best interests of the patient. Some of these patients with at best only partial bone marrow remissions have quite a good clinical remission and require little symptomatic support.

4. Supportive Measures

The therapist is committed to vigorous supportive measures if aggressive specific treatment is adopted. In general, a good remission is worth the hazards of cytotoxic drug therapy in acute leukaemia. Some complications of treatment are inevitable, and because supportive treatment plays such a prominent and important part in the management, special mention is made here.

Supportive measures are needed more for the complications of the drug treatment than of the disease itself. Anaemia and thrombocytopenia are often part of the disease and they may become temporarily worse after the cytotoxic drugs are given. Blood and platelet transfusions are usually required (Aisner, 1977).

The destruction of large quantities of leukaemic cells may precipitate excessive amounts of uric acid in the renal tubules and lead to renal failure. For this reason, allopurinol should be given routinely with the cytotoxic drug therapy, especially during induction and consolidation.

Another complication is the encephalopathy that may occur after intrathecal methotrexate and occasionally after cranial irradiation. Recovery is usual.

Infection is the greatest single hazard during the leucopenic phase, with septicaemia high on the list of infective complications (Steinberg, 1975). Gram-negative organisms, especially *Pseudomonas*, are among the first suspected when the patient develops a fever. Gentamicin and carbenicillin are prescribed on clinical diagnosis pending reports on cultures taken from multiple sites.

Non-bacterial infections are also common. Herpes simplex is a frequent, recurring, painful complication in patients with acute leukaemia. Monilial pharyngitis and oesophagitis are a common consequence of treatment. Stomatitis and ulcerations due to bacteria, viruses and drug therapy need appropriate attention. Herpes zoster is occasionally seen but is far more frequent in Hodgkin's disease and lymphomas. *Pneumocystis carinii* and cryptococcal infection may also complicate the picture.

Granulocyte transfusions are sometimes tried to combat repeated infections, particularly when the leucopenic phase is unduly prolonged. The real value of granulocyte transfusions remains in some doubt, large quantities of cells are needed and adverse reactions are not uncommon (Schiffer, 1977; Schimpff, 1977).

Methods of preventing infection have received considerable attention. Bowel sterilisation aims at eradicating one source of pathogens, topical antibiotics another (Storring et al., 1977). Isolation of the patient in a laminar air flow room or plastic tent is an effective prophylactic measure. Conventional barrier nursing also reduces the number of infective complications. Patients isolated for long periods tend to become mentally depressed and this aspect of support should not be overlooked.

The treatment of acute myeloblastic leukaemia and the complications of treatment can be very trying for the patient. Some clinicians advocate a less radical chemotherapeutic approach to the disease on the grounds of reducing the risk of life threatening adverse effects. Others hesitate to do so on the grounds that a safer compromise might reduce the chances of complete remission.

5. Conclusions

Acute lymphoblastic leukaemia of childhood responds well to vincristine and prednisone, with a survival of nearly 3 years in 50% of cases.

Acute myeloblastic leukaemia is treated with daunorubicin, cytarabine and many other drugs. The results of treatment are poor.

Supportive measures are an essential part of the management of acute leukaemia.

Chapter XIV

Chronic Leukaemias

1. Chronic Lymphocytic Leukaemia

1.1 Indications for Treatment

A few patients with chronic lymphocytic leukaemia remain well for maybe 10 years or longer without any apparent change in the nature of their disease, and may die from unrelated causes at a great age. The lymphocyte count in these cases remains constant at any level between $10{,}000/mm^3$ and $100{,}000/mm^3$.

Perhaps treatment should be commenced on diagnosis but rightly or wrongly, it is often prescribed only when patients have symptoms or develop signs of progressive disease. The same rule is rarely applied to a patient with indolent lymphocytic lymphoma. Curiously, a small lump is far more likely to evoke therapeutic enthusiasm than a load of 100,000 lymphocytes per cubic millimetre of blood.

Unfortunately, patients with the very chronic form of lymphocytic leukaemia or lymphoma are in the minority, and it will take many years to establish whether or not treatment converts a good prognosis into a better one.

If the plan of action is observation only, it is important to realise that symptoms may develop so insidiously that the patient is unaware of them. He may even deny symptoms when asked, attributing fatigue or lack of energy to his increasing age. Only in retrospect, after treatment, does he realise that his health was failing (Cridland, 1974).

The majority of patients have definite symptoms on diagnosis and require treatment. It is most often a disease of B lymphocytes, rarely of T lymphocytes, which carries a worse prognosis and responds less readily to treatment.

1.2 Methods of Treatment

An alkylating agent such as chlorambucil in relatively small doses is the basis of treatment. It is usually given in a series of courses with daily doses of about 0.1mg/kg, because responsive cases of chronic lymphocytic leukaemia are usually very sensitive to alkylating agents. Some prefer higher doses but caution should be observed because bone marrow function is impaired and megakaryocytes are often reduced.

In less than 5% the white cell and differential counts revert to normal. A good partial remission means relief of symptoms, a rise in haemoglobin, reduction in lymphocyte count and regression of enlarged nodes and spleen.

Corticosteroids are indicated in cases of anaemia and thrombocytopenia and those difficult to control with chlorambucil alone. If the patient has a haemoglobin of less than 10g/100ml prednisone should be given, alone at first, adding chlorambucil later when the haemoglobin has risen. The alkylating agent can also restore the haemoglobin level but recovery is quicker with steroids alone. A daily dose of 20 to 30mg usually suffices and high dose prednisone is not necessary except in more refractory cases of haemolytic anaemia. Corticosteroids cause a sudden rise in the white cell count which is no indication to alter treatment. The drug should be withdrawn when remission is achieved. In the more active forms of the disease, prednisone has to be used more freely.

At the beginning of treatment, blood counts should be done every 3 weeks or so. The frequency of subsequent counts depends upon the nature of the disease, the dose of alkylating agent given and the duration of the courses. In the past, many if not most patients were treated with low dose long term courses of chlorambucil without drug related complications. This method is still widely used although there is a trend towards a series of intermittent courses instead.

Some patients with chronic lymphocytic leukaemia are particularly prone to infection and they tend to have marked degrees of hypogammaglobulinaemia and neutropenia. Prolonged phases of drug induced neutropenia can add to the chances of infection and should be avoided.

Solar keratoses, which are very common in some countries such as Australia, may progress to squamous cell carcinomas which can behave in a most malignant way in patients with chronic lymphocytic leukaemia or lymphocytic lymphoma. All hyperkeratoses should therefore be treated promptly and if a squamous cell carcinoma is suspected it should be removed surgically as soon as possible. Radiotherapy is unsatisfactory in these particular cases.

While most patients benefit from treatment, there are a few for whom even partial remissions are not obtained. Other drugs, especially vincristine, are worth trying if a change in dose schedule of alkylating agents and prednisone fails, but the results with other drugs in the poor responders are disappointing (Desai et al., 1970).

Radiotherapy has a place in the management of chronic lymphocytic leukaemia. Large lymph node masses or a large spleen failing to regress satisfactorily after chemotherapy, may be irradiated. Lytic deposits in bone, an uncommon manifestation, are best treated with radiotherapy.

Splenectomy can bring benefit in selected cases of haemolytic anaemia, neutropenia or thrombocytopenia not controlled by other means.

The late stages of chronic lymphocytic leukaemia are often characterised by anaemia, while infection is a recurring problem and a frequent cause of death. Acute lymphoblastic leukaemia occurs very rarely. Only supportive measures are of any real value in end-stage disease (Galton, 1959; Galton, 1969; Silver, 1969).

2. Chronic Myelocytic Leukaemia

Unlike chronic lymphocytic leukaemia, the myelocytic form tends to be a relatively uniform disease in its natural history and its response to treatment.

The disease has a chronic phase of about 4 or 5 years' duration and an acute myeloblastic phase which responds poorly to all known forms of treatment. The phase of blastic transformation may lead to a fatal outcome in less than 6 months. In a few cases the later stage of the disease is characterised instead by anaemia, which is also refractory to treatment. The anaemic phase often terminates in myeloblastic transformation.

Most patients with typical signs of chronic myelocytic leukaemia have the abnormal Philadelphia chromosome. Those who lack this abnormality, about 5%, have a less favourable prognosis.

2.1 Indications for Treatment

By the time the disease is diagnosed, most patients have symptoms and require treatment. The alkylating agent busulphan has become the established drug of choice. Quite small doses are usually recommended, starting with 0.06mg/kg daily, and the initial course is continued for about 10 to 12 weeks in most cases. The drug is stopped when the white cell count is between 20,000/mm^3 and 10,000/mm^3 (fig. 2).

Further courses of busulphan are given when the disease begins to relapse, the aim being to keep the blood count normal or near normal. Complete clinical remission occurs in almost all cases, but complete bone marrow remission is not usually seen (Canellos, 1976; Galton, 1969).

In a few cases the count rises abruptly as soon as busulphan is suspended. To maintain remission the drug has to be given on a semi-continuous basis, a daily dose of 2mg or less usually sufficing to keep the count within normal limits. Treatment should also be designed to keep the platelet count within an acceptable range.

As previously mentioned, high doses of busulphan offer no therapeutic advantage and may be dangerous. It is known that the dose schedule originally described by Galton (1959) effectively reduces the tumour load in chronic myelocytic leukaemia. Cytokinetic studies have confirmed that the peripheral white cell count reflects the total granulocyte mass. The doubling time can be measured by plotting the white cell counts on a semilogarithmic scale, thus providing a convenient indication of the activity of the disease and the effect of treatment upon it (fig. 2).

Chronic myelocytic leukaemia has a relatively uniform natural history in the majority, but in a few cases the doubling time may be only 4 weeks and in others more than a year, so that a standardised maintenance dose schedule is not always applicable. Nevertheless, in spite of the orderly control that seems possible with busulphan, the treatment of chronic myelocytic leukaemia is far from ideal as it does not prevent blastic transformation.

Splenic irradiation is also a useful method of treatment, repeated for relapses. However, remissions are more easily sustained with chemotherapy, the haemoglobin level is kept consistently high and survival time is rather longer with busulphan than with radiotherapy (MRC, 1968).

Busulphan has a number of curious but uncommon side effects, notably bronzing of the skin and a wasting syndrome after long continued use. Intra-alveolar fibrosis is another side effect but one not necessarily related to long term use of busulphan. It is the complication most frequently sought, but not found, and seldom causes clinical problems. Other drugs such as melphalan can be used if these untoward effects of busulphan occur. Mitobronitol is another drug that has proved as effective as busulphan in the control of the disease. One trial comparing cyclophosphamide with busulphan showed busulphan more satisfactory in every respect (Kaung et al., 1971).

Treatment of the blastic transformation is rarely rewarding. Drugs such as mercaptopurine, vincristine, hydroxyurea, methotrexate, cytarabine, daunorubicin and adriamycin, either alone or in various combinations, are not often successful in inducing good remissions.

Sometimes the transition from the chronic to the myeloblastic phase is far from definite, with insidious onset of symptoms and very gradual clinical deterioration over several months. The patient may complain of fatigue or lack of energy. The haemoglobin falls a little and the percentage of immature granulocytes increases slightly in the peripheral count. The spleen may become palpable but bone marrow appearances remain unchanged without any evidence of impending blastic transformation. Busulphan is usually continued until there is certain evidence of the acute phase, but some advocate an earlier change to hydroxyurea or other class of drug. Occasionally the change reverses the deterioration, but occasionally too, the patient's condition improves again while continuing with busulphan. Presumably blastic change was not imminent.

Myeloblastic transformation is part of the natural history of the disease and appears to be neither induced nor prevented by treatment of the chronic phase. Occasionally patients present initially with this phase of the disorder.

Sometimes patients with chronic myelocytic leukaemia develop leukaemic infiltrations which may form quite large tumour masses, involve lymph nodes, or cause lytic lesions in bones. These are best treated with radiotherapy.

Infection, apart from that induced by over-zealous treatment, is not a feature of chronic myelocytic leukaemia. Overdosage from busulphan rarely results from conventional dose schedules. When the drug is continued too long after the count has fallen steeply towards 10,000/mm^3, pancytopenia may occur with its usual complications, and recovery is often slow.

3. Conclusions

Chronic lymphocytic leukaemia responds well to alkylating agents such as chlorambucil. Corticosteroids are useful for their lymphocytolytic effect and in some cases of anaemia associated with the disease.

Busulphan induces a complete clinical remission in most cases of chronic myelocytic leukaemia. The blastic transformation responds poorly to treatment.

Chapter XV

Hodgkin's Disease

Better methods of staging Hodgkin's disease have contributed greatly to improved results of treatment. Formerly, many patients treated with radiotherapy for stage I disease, had stage II, and many treated for stage II, had stage III, relapsing within 2 years or so. Patients were referred for chemotherapy only when the disease was far advanced. It is of interest that some patients formerly undertreated as stage I or II Hodgkin's disease could have long remissions in spite of having generalised disease from the outset.

In more recent years most of those treated appropriately with radiation therapy have true stage I or stage II Hodgkins' s disease, with a good chance of having all involved nodes irradiated and therefore a good chance of cure (Frei and Gehan, 1971; Johnson, 1969; Johnson et al., 1970; Kaplan, 1966; Kaplan, 1968; Perry et al., 1967; Peters et al., 1966). In stage III, remissions last 3 years or longer in up to 80% of cases, and there is a chance that many of these patients might also be cured. The importance of staging must therefore be emphasised (table IV) [Aisenberg and Goldman, 1970; De Vita and Carbone, 1971; Johnson et al., 1971; Lee and Spratt, 1974; Rapoport et al., 1969; Sahakian, 1975].

1. Indications for Chemotherapy

In some centres, stage III disease is also treated with radiotherapy and in selected cases this is the treatment of choice. Those with more extensive stage III disease and those with stage IV are usually better treated with chemotherapy initially (Gamble et al., 1973; Hoogstraten et al., 1973).

2. Methods of Treatment

High dose intermittent chemotherapy in the form of MOPP (mustine, Oncovin [vincristine], procarbazine and prednisone), developed by De Vita et al. (1970) is a

Table IV. Staging and treatment of Hodgkin's disease

Stage[1]	Description	Treatment[2]
I	Disease limited to one anatomical site	Radiotherapy
II	Disease limited to two anatomical sites on the same side of the diaphragm	Radiotherapy ± chemotherapy in stage IIB
III	Disease on both sides of the diaphragm, limited to lymph nodes, spleen and Waldeyer's ring	i) Chemotherapy ii) Radiotherapy in early stage III iii) Sequential chemotherapy and radiotherapy
IV	Disease also involving liver, lung, bone marrow and other tissues	Chemotherapy

1 All stages are subclassified; A: absence of systemic symptoms; B: presence of systemic symptoms.

2 The approach to treatment is also modified by the histopathological type of Hodgkin's disease.

most satisfactory method of management. Several similar combinations and dose schedules have proved equally effective (Bonadonna et al., 1977; Nicholson et al., 1970; Nissen et al., 1973). Six cycles of chemotherapy are given at intervals of 2 weeks.

Maintenance therapy in the form of a single cycle of MOPP, or other suitable agents, every 2 or 3 months has been shown in some series to prolong the disease-free period (Luce et al., 1973; Nissen et al., 1973), but maintenance therapy does not appear to increase the survival time. Continuing single cycles of treatment at selected intervals may be indicated for those in partial remission, but otherwise treatment is better withheld during remission to preserve the bone marrow for future chemotherapy when necessary (Young et al., 1973). Low dose maintenance chemotherapy should never be given in Hodgkin's disease.

It should not be overlooked that radiotherapy also has a place in the management of generalised Hodgkin's disease, either as part of the initial treatment or at any time during the course of the disease. Very large tumour masses are often best treated with radiotherapy, and symptoms such as pain from localised disease or bone deposits can be relieved rapidly by radiation therapy.

Radiotherapy and chemotherapy should not be given simultaneously because of the compounded effect on the blood count. If pancytopenia develops all treatment might have to be suspended for the time being. Exceptions include emergencies, such as superior vena caval obstruction or spinal cord compression. A single injection of mustine, 0.4mg/kg, is common practice at the commencement of radiotherapy for these emergencies in which rapid resolution of the tumour is necessary.

The value of prednisone in MOPP, COPP or other similar combinations for Hodgkin's disease is debatable. Given alone its effect is at best only transient. Although its inclusion can enhance the initial clinical response rate, giving a more rapid reduction of the ESR and temperature, without cytotoxic agents these benefits are not sustained. While there are few objections to its short term inclusion in MOPP, the long term use of prednisone has little place in the management of Hodgkin's disease except when there is haemolytic anaemia. Pruritus is occasionally most severe and intractable and a small dose of prednisone may bring some relief; unfortunately, however, the combination of steroids and scratching can lead to skin infection and more serious infective consequences.

MOPP can be repeated when the disease recurs. Extra care should be observed if the patient has had previous courses of chemotherapy or if extensive radiation therapy has destroyed bone marrow.

In spite of good results, there are patients who refuse to continue with MOPP therapy and the old and frail tolerate it poorly. There are several chemotherapeutic alternatives for these patients. A few might accept the rather less emetic COPP combination, but as a rule the therapeutic compromise must go further. The combination of chlorambucil and vinblastine is effective and has fewer side effects (Lacher and Durant, 1963). However, the dosage must be adequate to suppress Hodgkin's disease, and anti-emetics may still be needed. Vinblastine is given on day 1, with chlorambucil in high doses for 10 to 14 days, repeated at intervals of 2 to 4 weeks. Six cycles (including the cycles of MOPP already given) should suffice.

When Hodgkin's disease involves bone marrow to an appreciable extent, its response to chemotherapy is greatly impaired. Whereas lymphocytic infiltration is more sensitive to cytotoxic agents and can be readily cleared from the marrow in lymphocytic lymphoma, such is not the case in Hodgkin's disease. The relatively higher doses needed in Hodgkin's disease are hazardous in the presence of impaired bone marrow function. Treatment is difficult and this is one of the worst prognostic factors in the disease.

In late stage Hodgkin's disease, responding poorly to MOPP and similar combinations, other combinations which include drugs such as adriamycin, carmustine and dacarbazine may effect worthwhile partial remissions.

3. Conclusions

Most patients with stage III and stage IV Hodgkin's disease are treated with chemotherapy. High dose intermittent courses of a combination such as MOPP is the method of choice. Maintenance chemotherapy is not recommended for patients in complete remission.

Radiotherapy also has an important place in the management of generalised Hodgkin's disease.

Chapter XVI

Lymphomas

In generalised lymphoma chemotherapy is the treatment of choice although radiotherapy also has an important part to play (Stutzman, 1971). Some advocate that radiotherapy should take the major part in the management of selected cases (Johnson, 1972; Johnson et al., 1970a). As in Hodgkin's disease, large tumour masses, painful bone deposits, spinal cord compression and vena caval obstruction are among the indications for radiation treatment. If chemotherapy, including corticosteroids, fails to cause regression of lymphomatous masses or there is early recurrence after adequate drug therapy, radiotherapy is indicated.

An aggressive therapeutic approach may be taken with all cases of non-Hodgkin's lymphoma, whether they are of the rapidly progressive form of histiocytic lymphoma or the well differentiated type (Bonadonna and Monfardini, 1974; Carbone, 1972; Ultman, 1970). Certainly more vigorous chemotherapy has improved the results in some of the so-called histiocytic forms of the disease. It is essential to determine the optimal method of treatment. It is debatable whether a standardised chemotherapeutic policy is applicable to a disease with such a wide range of activity as non-Hodgkin's lymphoma.

At present there is a tendency to modify chemotherapy regimens, and the radiotherapeutic approach, to a greater extent in lymphoma than is usual in the treatment of Hodgkin's disease. The age of the patient, the sites of involvement and known activity of the disease, and the severity of bone marrow involvement are among the factors that influence the choice of treatment.

In children, and usually in young adults, lymphoma occurs in its less differentiated forms and is associated with a poor prognosis. A more radical attitude to initial treatment, as in acute leukaemia, is generally adopted.

1. Lymphocytic Lymphoma

The disease is one of the most sensitive to alkylating agents which are the drugs of choice and the basis of combination chemotherapy. Corticosteroids are also most useful in the management of lymphocytic lymphoma.

In well differentiated lymphocytic lymphoma, and the nodular variety in particular, remissions of many years can result from a single course of chlorambucil or even the irradiation of 2 or 3 anatomically separated lymph node regions. These forms of minimal treatment are now rarely applied, but the data illustrate how indolent the disease can be. The majority of patients with well differentiated disease have a good prognosis, and more active treatment aims at enhancing their survival and increasing the proportion of patients who survive longer than 10 years. There is still uncertainty about the optimal management of patients in this selected group. In some centres, 'total nodal' irradiation is favoured in the hope of prolonging remissions and survival in lymphocytic lymphoma (Johnson et al., 1970; Johnson, 1972).

The combinations COPP (cyclophosphamide, Oncovin [vincristine], procarbazine and prednisone) and COP (without procarbazine) are effective and the most popular. Six courses are usually given, either as originally prescribed or modified in dosage or dose schedule. Chlorambucil may be used instead of cyclophosphamide in the combination LOP (Leukeran [chlorambucil], Oncovin [vincristine] and prednisone). As an effective alternative, planned courses of either alkylating agent alone can be given (Cridland and Green, 1968; Ezdinli and Stutzman, 1965).

After initial courses of chemotherapy, the patients are usually observed, without maintenance treatment, then treated again on relapse. Remissions vary greatly in duration, from weeks to several years, so that the need for some form of maintenance therapy is likely to remain questionable for the time being. On the principle of keeping the malignant cell population at a minimum, it might be argued that a short series of intensive courses of treatment at selected intervals might effectively suppress recurrence. On the other hand, repeated treatment might only cause unwanted immunosuppression without eradicating 'quiescent' disease.

Corticosteroids are invaluable for their lymphocytolytic effect in lymphocytic lymphoma, and their ability to correct anaemia even when no direct evidence for haemolysis can be demonstrated. While long term use of prednisone should be avoided if possible, in some cases good remissions cannot be maintained without corticosteroids. Even as little as 10mg of prednisone daily may suffice. In several of the published dose schedules, prednisone dosage is very high, though short term. It is doubtful if daily doses of 100mg or more are of more value than 40mg or less in the vast majority of cases.

Caution with chemotherapy should be observed when megakaryocytes are reduced and the bone marrow is heavily infiltrated with lymphocytes. With care, however, even dense infiltration of the marrow can be cleared by chemotherapy.

Lymphocytosis in the peripheral count is seen regularly in about 10% of lymphocytic lymphomas, and frank lymphocytic leukaemia in up to 10% in older series; this is not necessarily a bad prognostic sign. Acute lymphoblastic change is an uncommon terminal manifestation of lymphocytic lymphoma. Vincristine and prednisone are the agents first tried, then others known to be useful in primary lymphoblastic leukaemia. The response to treatment is usually very poor.

Mediastinal node involvement is a prominent feature of Hodgkin's disease, but symptomatic pleural effusion tends to be a more frequent problem in non-Hodgkin's lymphoma. The cause of a pleural effusion is not always obvious so that a combination of cytotoxic drugs and prednisone is usually the treatment of choice. Irradiation of the mediastinum, and pleural deposits if present, may be an effective alternative.

Spinal cord compression and vena caval obstruction are managed in the same way as those complications in Hodgkin's disease with a combination of radiotherapy and chemotherapy. Rapid resolution of obstructing disease is essential, and in lymphomas prednisone assumes greater importance than in Hodgkin's disease in this regard.

When courses of treatment have been given in too high a dose or for too long, quite a long period of leucopenia may ensue, thus exposing the patient to infections to which he is already prone, irrespective of drug induced susceptibility. Infections commonly complicate the late stages but a few patients suffer from recurrent infection throughout the course of their disease, even in spite of remissions. Low concentrations of gamma globulins are the rule in these cases and neutropenia is a frequent accompaniment.

Other drugs such as adriamycin have a place in the control of progressive, relapsing disease not responding well to alkylating agents, vinca alkaloids and prednisone (Bonadonna and Monfardini, 1974). Whereas in late Hodgkin's disease, persistence with chemotherapy quite often achieves a good partial remission, in end-stage lymphoma the chances of success are less.

2. Histiocytic Lymphoma

2.1 Indications for Chemotherapy

Generalised disease due to so-called histiocytic lymphoma is an indication for chemotherapy and courses are often prescribed after irradiation of apparently localised disease.

In the nodular variety, with a mixed lymphocytic-histiocytic histology, the prognosis is better and the disease may even behave more like the lymphocytic lymphomas, with long complete remissions and long survival; in other cases it behaves like the more malignant diffuse type of histiocytic lymphoma. At diagnosis the prognosis is uncertain, but statistics support the case for a more vigorous approach to treatment (Bonadonna and Monfardini, 1974).

2.2 Methods of Treatment

High dose intermittent chemotherapy such as MOPP or COPP is used with good effect in many cases. It is nevertheless a fact that in spite of improved methods, many of the undifferentiated aggressive forms of lymphoma fail to respond well, even to aggressive therapeutic measures. The disease may be inherently resistant to chemotherapy and may respond poorly to radiotherapy as well. Histiocytic lymphomas may also display marked sensitivity to cytotoxic drugs and regress rapidly, only to recur before the bone marrow has recovered. Corticosteroids are of limited value in histiocytic lymphoma. If response to MOPP or COPP is poor, adriamycin and other drugs may be tried, although optimism is often unfounded. Continued poor response indicates a bad prognosis.

The disease has a tendency to infiltrate and cause pain. Radiotherapy is usually the treatment of choice when this occurs. Skin infiltrations, often raised purple tumours, are another characteristic. Radiotherapy may be used, but if the disease is widespread, which is more often the case, chemotherapy is the better method.

The recurrent, progressive form of the disease is difficult to treat, particularly when the bone marrow is involved. The picture is not unlike that of acute myeloblastic leukaemia, but the chances of bone marrow remission are remote. Even a good partial remission is a rare event.

3. Histiocytic Medullary Reticulosis

This rare disorder is usually rapidly fatal, and thought to be a variant of histiocytic lymphoma. Response to treatment is poor. There are isolated reports of satisfactory response to cytotoxic agents, corticosteroids and splenectomy.

4. Conclusions

Lymphocytic lymphoma responds well to alkylating agents and prednisone, often given in combination with vincristine. The extent of the disease and bone marrow impairment, and the age and condition of the patient may determine the type of chemotherapy prescribed in lymphocytic lymphoma. Maintenance therapy is not recommended during remission. Corticosteroids are useful in active forms of the disease.

Histiocytic lymphoma is best treated with combinations such as MOPP or COPP. It may respond poorly to all known forms of treatment. Radiotherapy also has a place in the treatment of generalised lymphoma, whether lymphocytic or histiocytic.

Chapter XVII

Mycosis Fungoides and Burkitt's Lymphoma

1. Mycosis Fungoides

Radiotherapy and chemotherapy are both useful in controlling the skin lesions and lymphomatous deposits in mycosis fungoides (Epstein et al., 1972). In reported series, 30 to 80% or more patients developed lymphoma during the course of mycosis fungoides.

The skin lesions are sometimes remarkably sensitive to quite small doses of alkylating agents. Complete resolution may occur after courses of chlorambucil 8 to 10mg daily. However, the sensitivity of the disease varies, and moderately high dose intermittent chemotherapy is recommended. Worthwhile remissions occur in about 50% of patients.

Chlorambucil, cyclophosphamide, mustine, procarbazine and vinblastine, with or without prednisone, are among the drugs shown to be useful and high dose methotrexate with folinic acid rescue can produce good results. Topical mustine and steroids have also been tried on more superficial lesions with some benefit.

Sezary's syndrome of generalised erythroderma might be a variant of mycosis fungoides and may respond to cytotoxic agents.

2. Burkitt's Lymphoma

Burkitt's lymphoma is potentially curable by chemotherapy in perhaps 40 to 50% of cases. Some of the long term survivors have had only a single dose of cyclophosphamide 40mg/kg, the dose shown to be effective more than 15 years ago (Clifford et al., 1967). However, several courses of combined chemotherapy are now recommended (Ziegler, 1972; Ziegler, 1977). A combination of radiotherapy and chemotherapy may offer the best chance of cure in some cases (Sturtz et al., 1972).

The response rate to cyclophosphamide or other drugs such as mustine, methotrexate or vincristine is 80%. Host defences are known to play an important part, and spontaneous remissions are occasionally seen.

Long term survival after treatment is influenced by the extent of the disease and the age of the patient, the young with localised disease having the best prognosis. In stage I and II disease the long term survival rate is about 70%, in stage III 50%, and in stage IV up to 45%.

Chapter XVIII

Multiple Myeloma, Plasmacytoma and Macroglobulinaemia

1. Indications for Treatment of Myeloma

Chemotherapy has increased survival time in myelomatosis. Most patients are treated on diagnosis. A few, particularly the 20% or so who have diffuse osteoporosis and no lytic bone lesions, have no symptoms. Opinion is divided on the need for these patients to be treated before signs and symptoms of progressive disease supervene.

Patients with typical multiple myeloma are often anaemic and have bone pain from deposits or pathological fractures. Some may even present with renal failure due to precipitation of Bence Jones protein in the tubules, or from secondary amyloidosis. Renal failure is usually a poor prognostic sign. Hypercalcaemia is another complication of multiple myeloma which may be among the presenting signs.

2. Methods of Treatment

Severe localised pain, commonly due to compression fractures of vertebrae, is usually best treated with radiation therapy which can relieve symptoms rapidly.

The alkylating agents are the basis of chemotherapeutic management of multiple myeloma. Melphalan, chlorambucil and cyclophosphamide have been widely used and appear to be equally effective (Alexanian et al., 1972; Costa et al., 1973; George et al., 1971; Rivers and Patno, 1969).

Probably the most popular schedule is a 5 day course of melphalan and prednisone at intervals of 6 weeks. Other drugs such as vincristine, adriamycin and

BCNU (carmustine) are sometimes used, more often in those cases which respond poorly to the above mentioned alkylating agents (Rosen, 1975). If the patient still has residual pain after chemotherapy, the affected region should be irradiated.

In all respects, short term intermittent chemotherapy in moderately high dosage is preferable to long term maintenance therapy, and the results are much better. There are exceptional cases, however, in which remission is better sustained by longer term treatment at low dosage.

At any time during the course of the disease, including the time of diagnosis, hypercalcaemia may develop. The patient must be immediately rehydrated and prednisone should be given. Cytotoxic drugs are withheld until hypercalcaemia is corrected and renal function is restored. Patients should be kept as mobile as possible.

Evaluation of results is rather unsatisfactory in myeloma. Worthwhile remissions are seen in at least 60%. Remissions are partial but may nevertheless be very good. Pain relief is often quite dramatic, even when x-ray appearances remain virtually unchanged. However, at least treatment can prevent or slow down progression of bone lesions. Bence Jones protein disappears early from the urine but the decrease in abnormal M-type serum globulins usually takes a few weeks. Effective treatment corrects anaemia although improvement in the bone marrow picture may not be readily demonstrated.

In some cases thrombocytopenia and leucopenia are a feature of the disease and more caution must be exercised in the use of cytotoxic drugs and the dose should be reduced.

Very rarely the disease terminates in plasma cell leukaemia, which does not respond well to treatment. Acute myeloblastic leukaemia is also rare but the reported incidence is increasing, possibly because more patients with myelomatosis now have a longer survival and are less likely to die from other complications.

Patients with myeloma are prone to infection, especially pneumonia. More intensive use of cytotoxic drugs and prednisone has led to an increased incidence of infection with Gram-negative organisms. Long intervals of drug induced leucopenia should be avoided to reduce the chances of serious infections.

3. Solitary Plasmacytoma

A localised tumour is treated by surgery and radiotherapy. In most cases of solitary tumour, the disease eventually becomes generalised, even years later. At that stage chemotherapy is indicated.

4. Macroglobulinaemia

When severe, and particularly when retinal vessels and renal function are threatened, plasmapheresis is done initially, before chemotherapy is commenced.

Long term courses of chlorambucil are often necessary to suppress the continuing activity of cells responsible for elaborating excessive amounts of M-type macroglobulins. Serial serum protein estimations provide a guide to the therapeutic progress. Prednisone is also a usual addition, especially when anaemia is a problem.

5. Conclusions

Courses of melphalan, chlorambucil or cyclophosphamide, combined with prednisone, are the treatment of choice for myeloma. Radiotherapy is often required for localised lesions.

Chapter XIX

Polycythaemia Vera and Myelofibrosis

1. Polycythaemia Vera

1.1 Indications for Treatment

It is in the best interests of the patient to maintain the haematocrit at 40 to 50% and platelet counts below 500,000/mm^3.

Treatment reduces the risk of the thrombotic and haemorrhagic complications of polycythaemia and thereby prolongs survival. Symptoms are at least largely relieved although persistence of some fatigue is common and may be due in part to iron deficiency.

1.2 Methods of Treatment

Venesection, phosphorus-32 and alkylating agents are employed in the control of the disease. Venesection is the most expedient means of reducing the red cell mass, and phosphorus-32 is probably still the most commonly applied method of suppressing the bone marrow activity (Dameshek, 1966; Watkins et al., 1967). Chemotherapy has the advantage of smoother control in this regard and it is used particularly in cases of severe thrombocytosis. A single dose of mustine, 0.4mg/kg IV can be given to reduce the platelet count quickly, and maintenance therapy may be added later.

Busulphan has been more widely accepted than other alkylating agents in polycythaemia vera, although reports of persistent thrombocytopenia after its long term administration have discouraged its use in more recent years. While thrombocytopenia is not a very common complication of busulphan treatment, chlorambucil or melphalan might be preferable alternatives.

There is no established chemotherapeutic schedule in polycythaemia vera. In some cases the platelet count can be kept within normal limits, together with some suppression of erythropoiesis, with an occasional course of busulphan or other agent. The duration of each course is determined by the response, but the average duration is about 8 to 10 weeks. There are cases, however, in which more prolonged and more frequent courses are required, especially in the initial stages. Most require only an occasional course of busulphan.

The interval between venesections and phosphorus-32 likewise varies according to the activity of the disease and remissions may last for weeks, months or many years.

If the patient with polycythaemia vera needs iron replacement after haemorrhage, only small amounts are required; recovery is rapid and if iron stores are restored to normal, haemopoietic activity will soon elevate the haematocrit to polycythaemic levels.

The late myelofibrotic phase of the disease is characterised by a progressive anaemia which responds poorly to specific treatment. The spleen also enlarges considerably. Chemotherapy has limited value at this stage but may reduce spleen size and relieve some symptoms. Radiotherapy is useful in relieving splenic pain. The acute leukaemia that may develop is a terminal manifestation for which treatment is rarely helpful.

1.3 Conclusions

Venesection, phosphorus-32 and busulphan are used to control polycythaemia vera. The late myelofibrotic and acute leukaemic stages of the disease respond poorly to treatment.

2. Myelofibrosis with Myeloid Metaplasia

2.1 Indications for Treatment

Myelofibrosis is best left untreated if symptoms are minimal. Troublesome constitutional symptoms and the discomfort of a large spleen are indications for treatment. A high platelet count should be reduced to lessen the risk of thrombosis.

2.2 Methods of Treatment

Chemotherapy is of limited value in this disease. Alkylating agents are the drugs of choice, busulphan in small doses being the one most commonly prescribed (Dameshek et al., 1958).

Constitutional symptoms of sweats, excessive fatigue and general weakness can in many cases be relieved, at least to some extent, by chemotherapy and pruritus is sometimes lessened. Chemotherapy should be used with the utmost caution in those with thrombocytopenia.

The spleen is often huge and even its partial reduction in size by the cautious use of busulphan or radiation therapy can bring symptomatic relief. Pain from splenic infarcts is readily relieved by radiotherapy. Reduction in spleen size may also result in a rise in the haemoglobin level if the spleen is the site of excessive red cell destruction. Corticosteroids are occasionally useful and the anaemia may respond to oxymetholone. Blood transfusions are given when the haemoglobin falls to intolerable levels.

The value of splenectomy remains a subject of perennial debate in the management of myelofibrosis. There are those who advocate removal of the spleen early in the course of the disease, while others prefer to delay until symptoms fail to respond to other forms of treatment. The consequences of splenectomy include gross enlargement of the liver and more marked thrombocytosis. On the other hand, splenectomy can be of great benefit to some patients.

The rare acute form of myelofibrosis responds poorly to all known forms of treatment.

2.3 Conclusions

Symptoms in myelofibrosis may be partially relieved by alkylating agents.

3. Primary Thrombocytosis

This is an uncommon syndrome that requires treatment only when the platelet count is persistently in excess of $500{,}000/mm^3$. An occasional course of an alkylating agent such as busulphan 2mg daily or less is usually adequate to keep the platelet count within normal limits.

Chapter XX

Carcinoma of the Breast

1. General Considerations

Cytotoxic drugs are indicated in clinically disseminated carcinoma of the breast and as adjunctive therapy for those patients whose disease is likely to recur.

Cytotoxic drugs cause regression of established clinical disease in about 50% of cases. The results are not good when the liver is known to be involved and are particularly poor when there are secondaries in the brain. Chemotherapy is a hazardous form of treatment when carcinoma cells have invaded the bone marrow.

The inadequacies of clinical staging make it difficult to plan appropriate treatment (Mansfield, 1976). True stage I and II cases are curable by surgery alone, but the actual extent of the disease cannot be determined with certainty at the time of operation. Most patients with breast cancer have metastatic disease at the time of diagnosis, either as detectable secondaries or as micrometastases (Cady, 1975; Fisher, 1977).

Survival correlates with the size of the operable primary, its histological type, the number of lymph nodes involved and the hormonal status of the patient (Cady, 1975). The most important single prognostic factor is lymph node involvement and those with fewer than 4 axillary nodes involved have a better prognosis than those with 4 or more affected. However, even in the absence of known metastases in axillary nodes, only some 75% of patients are alive and free of recurrence after 10 years (Fisher, 1977).

Not surprisingly, there is controversy over the need to use dangerous drugs when the chances of cure or long survival appear good (Leading Article, 1976). It is also argued that in the majority of cases recurrence is likely and that chemotherapy should be given early when metastatic foci are small (Bonadonna et al., 1976; Carter, 1976; Fisher, 1977; Fisher et al., 1975).

In spite of the fallacies of clinical staging and the many variables that complicate interpretation of results, useful information has emerged from clinical trials of adjuvant chemotherapy, and further trials are in progress. Most include patients under 75 years of age who have had radical mastectomy for potentially curable disease in which one or more axillary nodes were involved.

Short term observations have established that chemotherapy can prolong the so-called disease-free interval between primary treatment and recurrence. The figures also show that adjuvant chemotherapy can reduce the mortality rate in the first 2 years. It remains doubtful whether chemotherapy prolongs the average survival in breast cancer, but its effect on the survival of selected groups of responders is more relevant (Fisher, 1977).

Mansfield (1976) has summarised the problems of evaluating the various modes of treatment, with emphasis on surgery and radiotherapy. While it remains impossible to determine the true extent of breast cancer, optimal methods of treatment cannot be clearly defined. Mansfield's review of the literature also highlights the difficulty of comparing one series with another. There are many variables, quite apart from the variable nature of the disease itself. These include the proportions of pre- and postmenopausal patients in the different series; some have had ovarian, adrenal or pituitary ablation while others have not had even hormone therapy; surgical methods differ; some have had radiotherapy, others not.

Obviously it is not an isolated question of determining the value of chemotherapy in breast cancer. The contribution of chemotherapy is only part of the total management which itself has yet to be defined satisfactorily.

2. Methods of Chemotherapy

Moderately high doses of cytotoxic drugs are required in cancer of the breast. Alkylating agents alone, such as a 5 day course of melphalan every 6 weeks, or some similar schedule, has been used with good response in 30 to 70% (Carter, 1976; Carter and Livingston, 1975; Fisher et al., 1975). Bonadonna et al. (1976), have used more vigorous treatment, not only with higher dosage but also with more intensive dose schedules. They advocate a 3-drug combination of cyclophosphamide, methotrexate and fluorouracil (CMF). Less depilatory triple therapy with thiotepa, methotrexate and fluorouracil is an effective alternative. Quadruple therapy which includes vincristine or vinblastine is also widely used (Broder and Carbone, 1976; Carter and Livingston, 1977; Fisher, 1977; Haskell, 1977).

The dosage for each drug varies a little from one regimen to another, and the intervals between courses may also differ from once a week initially then every 6 weeks, or more commonly, a course every 3 or 4 weeks from the beginning. The interval is also altered whenever there is evidence of undue bone marrow depression. In the case of adjuvant therapy for those without known metastases, treatment is continued for 12 months to 2 years. If the disease recurs during the course, either a different drug combination or radiotherapy is given, whichever is appropriate. Patients with established metastatic disease are treated until there is failure of response.

If alkylating agents, vinca alkaloids, fluorouracil and methotrexate fail to control the disease there are other drugs and combinations known to have some effect. Adriamycin in particular, is active against carcinoma of the breast and is commonly combined with vincristine. The nitrosoureas are known to be useful in a minority and many other cytotoxic drugs have been shown to have some effect but are yet to be evaluated.

Radiotherapy retains an important place in the management of disseminated disease. All too often, pain from one or more bone deposits is not relieved by chemotherapy, and radiotherapy is then indicated.

Host defences are a factor in the prognosis of carcinoma of the breast. There have been several trials to suggest that chemo-immunotherapy may be better than chemotherapy alone, but this combined method of treatment is still experimental (Gutterman et al., 1976; Haskell, 1977).

The optimal chemotherapeutic schedule is yet to be worked out and in the case of 'prophylactic' treatment, weighed against the possible serious adverse effects associated with long term cancer chemotherapy.

3. Conclusions

Chemotherapy is indicated in disseminated carcinoma of the breast and in cases in which disease is expected to recur. Combinations of alkylating agents, vinca alkaloids, fluorouracil and methotrexate have proved to be effective. Chemotherapy can prolong the disease-free interval between primary treatment and recurrence.

Chapter XXI

Bronchogenic Carcinoma

Bronchogenic carcinoma is among the least sensitive to chemotherapy, with favourable responses uncommon and achieved mainly in cases of small cell carcinoma. In this type, significant progress has been made in the chemotherapeutic management using 3-drug combinations. Cyclophosphamide, methotrexate and lomustine (CCNU) achieved relatively good results with a complete remission rate of 25% (Bunn et al., 1973).

Probably every cytotoxic drug in clinical use has been tried in this disease. Relatively large doses are needed to evoke any measure of response and remissions are of short duration. The alkylating agents are among the most useful and are usually included in combination therapy. Of the single drugs, mustine and cyclophosphamide in high doses are the two most generally given. Methotrexate with folinic acid rescue, procarbazine, busulphan, the nitrosoureas and adriamycin have been used in quite large series and reported to have some effect in 15 to 30% of cases. Somewhat more favourable results have been reported with the combined use of a variety of drugs but so far combination chemotherapy has been predictably disappointing (Hansen, 1977).

Immunotherapy combined with chemotherapy has prolonged survival in a few cases (Gutterman et al., 1976), or improved the short term results (McKneally et al., 1976).

Palliative radiotherapy, though unsatisfactory, is a better form of treatment for inoperable or recurrent bronchogenic carcinoma, except in the small cell type.

Chapter XXII

Malignant Disease of the Genitourinary System

1. Ovarian Carcinoma

1.1 Indications for Chemotherapy

Chemotherapy is indicated in cases of inoperable or recurrent carcinoma of the ovary and for those patients who have, or probably have, residual disease after surgery. Cytotoxic drugs are therefore indicated in advanced stage II as well as stage III and IV disease.

Unfortunately, most patients with ovarian carcinoma have clinically advanced disease at the time of diagnosis and many have occult spread beyond the apparent sites involved. The 5-year survival for all patients with apparent stage I treated by surgery alone ranges from 32 to 78% in different series (Bagley et al., 1972).

Survival correlates with the stage of the disease (table V) and it is also influenced by the histological type and grade of malignancy. These factors determine the therapeutic plan, but even with improved methods, staging is not accurate (Anderson and Young, 1977).

Ovarian carcinoma responds well to alkylating agents in 50% of cases. About 50% are also radio-sensitive but not necessarily the same 50% of patients who respond well to chemotherapy. In general terms, when disease is apparently confined to the pelvis, a course of radiotherapy is usually the treatment of choice. When the disease is more widespread, and in older patients who might not tolerate radiotherapy well, chemotherapy is preferred after surgery. Chemotherapy is also given to those who have already had radiotherapy for inoperable or residual disease.

1.2 Methods of Treatment

The alkylating agents are the drugs of choice, chlorambucil, cyclophosphamide, melphalan and thiotepa being the most commonly used, all with an average response

Table V. Staging of primary carcinoma of the ovary

Stage and sub-category		Description
I		Tumour limited to ovaries
	Ia	Limited to one ovary i) capsule intact on external surface ii) tumour through capsule to external surface
	Ib	Tumour limited to both ovaries i) capsule intact on external surface ii) tumour through capsule to external surface
	Ic	Stage Ia or Ib and ascites with malignant cells in the fluid
II		Tumour of one or both ovaries with pelvic extension
	IIa	Extension to uterus or tubes
	IIb	Extension to other pelvic tissues
	IIc	Stage IIa or IIb and ascites with malignant cells in the fluid
III		Tumour involving one or both ovaries with intraperitoneal metastases outside the pelvis and/or involved retroperitoneal nodes Disease limited to true pelvis with extension to small bowel or omentum
IV		Tumour of one or both ovaries with distant metastases beyond the peritoneal cavity

rate of 50%. The disease may also be responsive to other drugs such as fluorouracil, methotrexate, vincristine, vinblastine and adriamycin, with response rates ranging from 10 to 30% (Anderson and Young, 1977; Bagley et al., 1972; Malkasian, 1974). Intracavity administration of drugs for effusion offers no advantage over the oral or intravenous route.

Combination chemotherapy appears not to be superior to alkylating agents alone (Bagley et al., 1972; Buchler et al., 1974; Malkasian, 1974), with the possible exception of the uncommon granulosa cell and Sertoli Leidig cell tumours (Schwartz and Smith, 1976). More recently, however, improved results have been reported with combination therapy in a number of series (Anderson and Young, 1977); the contribution of dose, dose schedule and better staging has yet to be assessed.

Progesterone compounds are reported to have some value in the treatment of carcinoma of the ovary but have not yet undergone adequate trials (Malkasian, 1974).

Irradiation of the abdomen after courses of chemotherapy did not prolong survival in a series of patients treated by Johnson et al. (1972). However, irradiation of a residual mass still present after chemotherapy may effect complete regression, and courses of chemotherapy for residual disease after radiotherapy can be similarly successful.

When recurrent disease fails to respond to further treatment with alkylating agents, the choice is radiotherapy or other types of cytotoxic drugs. If the recurrence is relatively localised, radiotherapy is preferred unless the region has already received full doses of radiation. Other drugs known to be effective, notably fluorouracil or methotrexate should be tried. Resistant recurrences may also respond well to platinum diamminodichloride (Gottlieb and Drewinko, 1975).

1.3 The Place of Prophylactic Chemotherapy in Ovarian Carcinoma

When cure has probably been achieved by surgery in stage Ia disease, that is, tumour confined to one ovary, neither radiotherapy nor chemotherapy is indicated. The chances of cure are good with a cure rate up to 90% if the tumour has not penetrated through the capsule (Anderson and Young, 1977). The risk of adverse effects from chemotherapy, including the higher incidence of acute leukaemia reported by Rivers et al. (1977), is a deterrent to the use of alkylating agents when the probability of cure by surgery alone is so high.

The place of radiotherapy, and certainly of chemotherapy, remains uncertain in stage Ib in which tumour involves both ovaries or in Ic when ascites is present. Postoperative radiotherapy improves the outlook in stage II, and it is common practice to prescribe a series of courses of chemotherapy on completion of radiotherapy.

The duration of 'prophylactic' chemotherapy is influenced by the relative risk of recurrence. For the majority the risk is high, and courses of treatment are given for about 2 years or until relapse. For the minority of patients with the greater likelihood of cure, treatment with cytotoxic drugs is stopped after about 18 months.

1.4 Dose Schedules

The optimal dose schedule for induction and maintenance of remission is not known. Response rates range from 30% to more than 60% with a variety of regimens. Some advocate long term low dose continuous therapy with an alkylating agent after the initial loading dose. While a few carcinomas of the ovary are exceptionally sensitive to chemotherapy, probably most require moderately high doses to effect regression. For this and other reasons, low dose maintenance therapy is not recommended.

Moderately high dose intermittent chemotherapy with an alkylating agent is preferable, but it is yet to be established how this should be scheduled. A series of 6 short courses at intervals of 2 or 3 weeks, then a course every 6 to 12 weeks is an effective method. Alternatively, regular courses every 4 to 6 weeks may be given. A series of 3 or 4 courses every few months after an initial 6 courses might be a better way of keeping the malignant cell population at a minimum.

Some form of intermittent maintenance therapy is indicated in the hope of improving the prognosis in advanced cases of ovarian carcinoma. In spite of long remissions in many instances, there have been reports of a tendency for the disease to recur if treatment is suspended for long. Furthermore, in stage III and IV, survival figures decline after 2 years, falling to 10% or less at 5 years.

While attempts to work out the optimal method with alkylating agents continue, further trials with combination therapy are in progress. A schedule such as MOPP deserves more attention. Combinations of other drugs are being applied in those cases resistant to alkylating agents, and these include not only recurrent resistant tumours, but also some 40% at diagnosis.

2. Testicular Tumours

These include seminoma, teratocarcinoma, embryonal carcinoma and choriocarcinoma, each with different sensitivities to cytotoxic drugs. Consistently good results are seen only in seminoma.

2.1 Seminoma

Radiotherapy is the treatment of choice because disseminated disease is still potentially curable.

In metastatic or recurrent disease beyond the scope of radiotherapy, alkylating agents are the drugs of choice, and they are often given in combination with other effective drugs such as vincristine. The response rate is 50 to 60%.

2.2 Embryonal Carcinoma, Choriocarcinoma and Teratocarcinoma

Courses of mithramycin have proved to be effective in embryonal carcinoma, with less success seen in the case of either choriocarcinoma or teratocarcinoma (Kuhbock et al., 1974). There are reports of response in up to 70% in embryonal carcinoma and a 15 to 30% complete remission rate, sometimes of several years' duration (Kennedy, 1974).

Mithramycin has also been used sequentially with actinomycin D, adriamycin and vinblastine. Chlorambucil and actinomycin D and later methotrexate, have been used in combination for many years in teratocarcinoma. Actinomycin D is thought by many to be the best single drug for testicular tumours, except for seminoma, but this impression might be due to longer experience in its use.

Other effective combinations include chlorambucil, actinomycin D and methotrexate with the addition of vincristine in some series. Courses of quadruple therapy with vincristine, fluorouracil, cyclophosphamide and methotrexate is another combination in current use. The dual combination of bleomycin with either vinblastine or lomustine (CCNU), or actinomycin D with mithramycin is also used in testicular tumours (Holoye and Samuels 1974; McElwain et al., 1974).

The platinum coordination complexes, known to have an adverse effect on sperm production in rats, are also active against testicular tumours. Platinum diamminodichloride has proved to be effective in up to 80 % of cases, including those failing to respond to other drugs such as actinomycin D. In view of its toxicity, the drug has a more useful place in combined regimens with other well tried drugs (Gottlieb and Drewinko, 1975; Hill et al., 1975).

3. Carcinoma of the Uterus

Progestagens and radiotherapy are of more value than cytotoxic drugs in disseminated endometrial carcinoma.

The alkylating agents, fluorouracil and adriamycin have been used with little success (Donovan, 1974). Combination chemotherapy is unlikely to improve the results greatly.

4. Carcinoma of the Cervix Uteri

Radiation therapy is the method of choice in recurrent or inoperable carcinoma of the cervix.

Alkylating agents and most other classes of cytotoxic drug have a consistently poor record in the treatment of this disease. The combination of bleomycin and methotrexate, however, is proving useful.

5. Gestational Choriocarcinoma

Chemotherapy is indicated in all cases of gestational choriocarcinoma because it is potentially curable. Untreated the disease is usually fatal within 12 months.

Chemotherapy is also given in cases of chorio-adenoma destruens and in hydatidiform mole if gonadotrophin levels rise.

Methotrexate has remained the drug of choice through the years although excellent results have been reported with many drugs including mustine, thiotepa, chlorambucil, cyclophosphamide, mitomycin, mercaptopurine and actinomycin D. Relatively high doses are required, and adequate supportive measures are essential (Condit, 1971; Hammond and Parker, 1970; Herz et al., 1965).

A number of dose schedules and combinations have been used with varying success. Repeated 5-day courses of methotrexate, a combination of methotrexate and mercaptopurine, the sequential or concurrent use of chlorambucil and actinomycin D, or methotrexate and actinomycin D have been recommended. Treatment is continued until gonadotrophin levels are persistently normal.

Opinion is divided on the value of radiotherapy, but on the whole, reported results have not been favourable.

6. Carcinoma of the Kidney

Hypernephroma (Grawitz tumour) is not noted for its sensitivity to cytotoxic drugs, although few have in fact been evaluated in the treatment of the tumour. Nevertheless, there have been only occasional reports of partial remissions and the results so far have not been encouraging.

Progestational hormones are of more palliative value (Bloom and Wallace, 1964).

7. Carcinoma of the Bladder

Poor results with chemotherapy are usual in carcinoma of the bladder. Attempts with high dose cyclophosphamide were not rewarding. Controlled trials with fluorouracil failed to support claims in earlier reports. At present adriamycin is the drug of promise in bladder carcinoma, and indeed in many other carcinomas.

Carcinoma of the bladder has not been the subject of many chemotherapy trials, either with single drugs or combination therapy. There is possibly some scope for improvement.

8. Carcinoma of the Prostate

Cytotoxic drugs have not been used extensively in disseminated prostatic cancer but a number of trials with combination therapy are in progress. The drugs most commonly tried are cyclophosphamide, fluorouracil and adriamycin, but the results so far have not been good. Moreover, in the advanced stages, bone marrow function may be impaired, placing limitations on the effective use of chemotherapy.

Hormone therapy remains the best form of palliation.

9. Nephroblastoma (Wilms' Tumour)

Radiotherapy after surgical removal then courses of chemotherapy is the method of management. Improved surgical and radiotherapeutic techniques increased the survival from 10% to about 50%, and the addition of chemotherapy improved the cure rate to some 80%.

Actinomycin D has had a place in the treatment of nephroblastoma for many years. Its value in the prevention of metastases as well as in treatment of established secondary disease was reported by Farber in 1966. There have since been reports of better results when actinomycin D is combined with vincristine. Treatment is given intermittently at intervals of 2 or 3 months for a period of 2 years after surgery and radiotherapy (Schwartz, 1977).

The tumour is sensitive to many different cytotoxic drugs such as mustine, cyclophosphamide, daunorubicin, adriamycin and carmustine (BCNU), and these should be tried if there is poor response or rapid recurrence. Even in cases of widely disseminated disease, chemotherapy and radiotherapy can achieve worthwhile results.

10. Conclusions

Ovarian carcinoma responds well to alkylating agents in 50% of cases. High dose intermittent chemotherapy is the method of choice.

Among testicular tumours, seminoma responds well to alkylating agents. Several types of cytotoxic drug are effective against embryonal carcinoma.

Carcinoma of the uterus, cervix, kidney, bladder and prostate respond poorly, if at all, to chemotherapy.

Chemotherapy has an established place in the management of gestational choriocarcinoma and nephroblastoma.

Chapter XXIII

Carcinoma of the Digestive System

1. Carcinoma of the Oesophagus

Surgery and radiotherapy have not yet produced good results and so far chemotherapy has less to offer. Bleomycin proved to be disappointing. The alkylating agents, though still included in some of the combined regimens, have also given poor results in the past. Some benefit has been observed after treatment with lomustine (CCNU) but the results are not impressive (Moertel, 1976).

2. Carcinoma of the Stomach

Most cytotoxic agents have been tried in recurrent gastric carcinoma but none so far has been really effective. Occasional good results have been reported with fluorouracil, one of the most widely used in this disease. Better responses have been achieved with fluorouracil combined with a nitrosourea, and more recently there have been quite promising reports on the use of adriamycin with carmustine (BCNU). However, remissions are partial and of short duration (Moertel, 1976).

3. Colorectal Carcinoma

Cyclophosphamide and fluorouracil have been popular drugs in attempts to treat recurrent colorectal cancer. Many different combinations have been tried with limited success. A combination of streptozocin, lomustine (CCNU), bleomycin, thioguanine and procarbazine among others, has given short remissions.

The results in colorectal carcinoma are somewhat better than those seen in other forms of gastrointestinal carcinoma (Heal and Schein, 1977). Colorectal carcinoma, however, can be slowly evolving. Even with liver metastases, 33% of patients survive 12 months, and 14% are still alive at 2 years with no treatment.

4. Secondary Carcinoma of the Liver

Liver involvement by metastatic carcinoma of the breast has a poor prognosis, but remissions with marked reduction in liver size, the size of tumours on scanning, and the disappearance of jaundice are sometimes obtained with combination chemotherapy. Triple or quadruple therapy with thiotepa or cyclophosphamide and fluorouracil, methotrexate and vinblastine is the usual combination.

Secondaries from the gastrointestinal tract are less responsive to systemic chemotherapy. Cyclophosphamide in high doses effects a few responses, similarly with fluorouracil or combinations of agents. The results have been more encouraging with regional arterial infusion with fluorouracil or methotrexate through the hepatic artery. Response rates up to 60% and more have been reported in cases of metastatic carcinoma of the colon. In one series, the quality of life was improved for these patients and the survival time increased by a few months. On the other hand, in one quite typical series, survival after hepatic artery infusions was little better than in untreated controls (Oberfield, 1975).

5. Hepatoma

Chemotherapy, systemic and by infusion, has been tried in hepatoma with reported response rates of 0 to 50% in small series, usually less than 10 patients.

Partial remissions have been obtained with fluorouracil, methotrexate and prednisone or a combination of bleomycin and adriamycin. The combined administration of fluorouracil and carmustine (BCNU) or fluorouracil and mitomycin is claimed to have more value (Oberfield, 1975).

6. Carcinoma of the Pancreas

Chemotherapy has a poor record in the treatment of carcinoma of the pancreas. At present adriamycin is thought to be the best in a long list of unsuccessful drugs. Islet cell carcinoma shows some response to chemotherapy.

7. Conclusions

Chemotherapy has some value in colorectal carcinoma.

The results are poor in carcinoma of the oesophagus, stomach, liver and pancreas.

Chapter XXIV

Miscellaneous Tumours

1. Osteosarcoma

High dose methotrexate with folinic acid 'rescue' is given in an attempt to prevent metastases and to control known secondaries. Intermittent 'prophylactic' chemotherapy is continued for the 2 year period in which metastatic disease is expected to occur (Jaffe, 1974; Jaffe, 1974a).

The tumour is not notably sensitive to cytotoxic drugs but objective response is seen after treatment with methotrexate and others. Methotrexate is often combined with vincristine, or with vincristine, adriamycin and cyclophosphamide. Dacarbazine is included in some regimens (Chang, 1977).

2. Ewing's Sarcoma

Some of the chemotherapeutic methods used in osteogenic sarcoma are also applied in cases of Ewing's sarcoma, with more success. The drugs used include cyclophosphamide, vincristine, actinomycin D and adriamycin. In one series a combination of vincristine, cyclophosphamide and carmustine (BCNU) was given (Schajowicz et al., 1974). There have been a few reports to suggest that chemotherapy as a 'prophylactic' measure after radiotherapy might improve the survival rate.

3. Soft Tissue Sarcomas

Local recurrence is a major problem in soft tissue sarcomas after surgery and high dose radiation therapy. Chemotherapy is therefore given in the hope of preventing recurrence as well as being of some value in the control of disseminated disease. Chemotherapy is also used initially in otherwise inoperable cases of rhabdomyosarcoma.

Actinomycin D, cyclophosphamide and vincristine in sequence, or more often in combination, are used. There have been a few encouraging results reported in cases of childhood rhabdomyosarcoma treated weekly for 6 weeks, then every 2 weeks for 12 months or longer (Donaldson et al., 1973; Malpas et al., 1974). Other soft tissue sarcomas, such as fibrosarcoma or liposarcoma are less likely to respond.

Adriamycin and dacarbazine are quite effective in about 30% of some soft tissue tumours, and used together have increased the response rate to about 60%. Similar results have been claimed with other combinations including cyclophosphamide, vincristine and methotrexate. This combination therapy is generally given in 5-day courses every 3 weeks (Benjamin et al., 1977).

4. Neuroblastoma

Chemotherapy is indicated when the disease is disseminated or there is residual tumour after surgery and radiotherapy. So far the use of 'prophylactic' chemotherapy has not increased the cure rate.

The overall response rate is 60% in most series, 25% being complete remissions with an average duration of 6 to 8 months. Although survival is longer among those patients who respond well, the overall survival rate has not been improved by chemotherapy (Evans et al., 1969; Schwartz, 1977).

Cyclophosphamide and vincristine either sequentially or concurrently have been well tried with quite good results. Adriamycin has proved to be a useful addition in improving the duration of remission. Other drugs such as chlorambucil, actinomycin D, methotrexate, daunorubicin and dacarbazine may also cause regression of the tumour.

Dose schedules differ from series to series. As an example, vincristine may be given every other week alternating with cyclophosphamide, continuing for 3 months, or longer if the response is good. Combination chemotherapy with 3 or 4 drugs is usually given in 5-day courses every month.

5. Retinoblastoma

This is a relatively sensitive tumour and recurrent disease may respond well to vincristine alone. However, vincristine is usually given in combination with such agents as fluorouracil, cyclophosphamide and methotrexate.

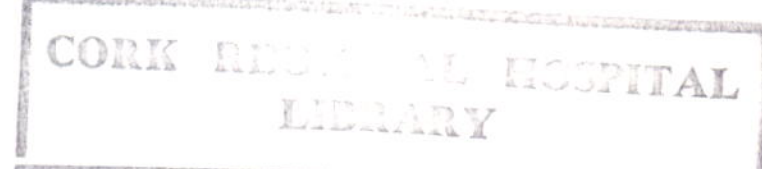

6. Melanoma

Melanoma responds poorly to chemotherapy. Complete regression has been observed occasionally after perfusion or infusion for localised disease (Krementz et al., 1974), but treatment of metastatic melanoma holds little reward. Immunotherapy with BCG seems to prolong remissions and reduce the incidence of early metastases (Morton et al., 1976). It is difficult to assess the value of chemotherapy in delaying recurrence or prolonging life in recurrent disease because melanoma can be so unpredictable.

Of the alkylating agents, melphalan has been well tried as a perfusion drug and as oral treatment, the latter without much benefit. A derivative of colchicine was reported as useful in a few cases. As might be expected, a wide variety of drugs either alone or in combination has been tried in melanoma. These include the alkylating agents, the nitrosoureas, vincristine, cytarabine and other pyrimidine analogues, all without remarkable success. The relatively new drug, dacarbazine has shown greater promise with a reported response rate of 24%. Combined with vincristine and carmustine (BCNU) in one series, the results were more encouraging.

Chemotherapy in melanoma is far from satisfactory (Cady, 1975a; Lichtenfield, 1977).

7. Brain Tumours

In the early trials of mustine slight relief of symptoms from cerebral metastases was observed in a few cases (Karnofsky, 1958). Perfusions or infusions with various agents, either alone or in combination, have also given discouraging results in both primary and secondary brain tumours (Walker, 1977).

The lipid soluble nitrosoureas on the other hand, can cross the blood-brain barrier in therapeutic concentrations. Marked benefit occurs in some cases, but the results are variable. In one series the survival figures in glioma were better when carmustine (BCNU) was added to the usual treatment with surgery and radiotherapy (Shapiro, 1974). In another series the addition of either carmustine or lomustine (CCNU) made no significant difference (Crivelli et al., 1974).

8. Carcinomatosis, Primary Unknown

Anaplastic malignant disease can present itself with widespread metastatic deposits in skin, lung, bone and other organs and the primary site may be unknown. As far as treatment is concerned, chemotherapy has little to offer.

Occasionally, multiple metastases turn out to be a histiocytic lymphoma which may respond well to chemotherapy (see page 63). Uncommonly they are due to ovarian carcinoma which may likewise be readily treatable (page 77). Usually, however, carcinomatosis has its origin in tumours not sensitive to chemotherapeutic agents, such as bronchogenic carcinoma, carcinoma of the stomach or pancreas and even melanoma, which may behave as an anaplastic, disseminated disease.

Palliative radiotherapy is more often the treatment of choice. Pain from bone deposits can be relieved, and partial regression of metastases in lung and other organs can bring at least symptomatic benefit.

Various drugs or combinations of drugs such as alkylating agents, vinca alkaloids, methotrexate, fluorouracil or adriamycin may be worth trying, provided the patient is not too inconvenienced. Patients must be carefully selected for chemotherapy. There is rarely justification for a morbidity rate in the treatment of carcinomatosis. Chemotherapy is hazardous when the bone marrow is involved.

In assessing the indications for treatment and its value in cases of widespread carcinoma, it is worthy of mention that a few patients may survive perhaps a year or more in quite good condition, without treatment.

9. Conclusions

Chemotherapy has a limited place in the treatment of malignant bone disease. Some soft tissue tumours respond to a number of cytotoxic agents. Occasional benefit is seen in melanoma and the nitrosoureas have some value in the management of brain tumours.

Carcinomatosis is usually due to tumours relatively insensitive to chemotherapeutic agents.

Chapter XXV

Immunotherapy

Immunotherapy, though old in concept, is only just emerging as a practical form of treatment for malignant disease. Alone, immunotherapy has had limited therapeutic impact, but in conjunction with cytotoxic drugs as immunochemotherapy, it has somewhat more potential.

Immunotherapy can be broadly classified as active, passive or adoptive. It may be specific or nonspecific. Adoptive immunotherapy with immune lymphocytes has met with limited success in man but bone marrow transplantation has been more successful. Passive immunotherapy with antitumour specific antibodies has obvious technical difficulties in the production of those antibodies, while experimental studies with antisera have yielded poor results. Serology as a practical method remains virtually confined to experimental tumours with antigenicity.

Active immunotherapy, by stimulating immune mechanisms to reject a tumour, shows more promise as an adjunct to cytotoxic drug and radiation therapy. A growing number of agents, called immunomodulators, have been utilised in this way. Early clinical work was done by Mathe in the treatment of childhood acute lymphoblastic leukaemia. After reducing the number of leukaemic cells with cytotoxic agents, attempts were made to destroy the residual cells by nonspecific stimulus with BCG and later with irradiated allogenic leukaemic cells. Improved results with BCG immunotherapy have been achieved more consistently in acute myeloblastic leukaemia and the addition of active specific immunotherapy with irradiated cells can increase survival still further. Many trials of this kind are still in progress (Hersh et al., 1976; Heyn et al., 1973; Mathe, 1969; MRC, 1971; Powles, 1976).

Malignant melanoma has been subjected to immunochemotherapy for several years. A combination of BCG and chemotherapy has improved the remission rate and also prolonged survival in some cases (Morton et al., 1976). In carcinoma of the breast there have been reports of longer remissions with immunochemotherapy compared with chemotherapy alone. Some results have suggested the superiority of immunochemotherapy in squamous cell carcinoma of the head and neck and possibly also in colorectal cancer (Gutterman et al., 1976).

There are hazards associated with BCG immunotherapy. An anaphylactic reaction, liver toxicity and a number of systemic symptoms are well documented. Local skin reactions are usually minimal and systemic infection is rare (Sparks, 1976; Sparks et al., 1973).

Corynebacterium parvum is another agent used for stimulating the production of antibody to several antigens. The organism activates macrophages and has been shown to enhance resistance to some infections in mice and to inhibit the growth of some animal tumours. *C. parvum* has been tried, with cytotoxic drug therapy, against a variety of malignant diseases in man and the results so far have warranted further clinical trials. *C. parvum* causes local reactions, some constitutional symptoms and, very occasionally, thrombocytopenia and renal toxicity (Oettgen et al., 1976).

Levamisole, a synthetic anthelminthic drug, also enhances the immune response (Oettgen et al., 1976). It has been reported to activate, and increase, antibodies to influenza vaccine and to have a number of stimulating effects on lymphocytes. Enhanced phagocytosis has been observed after levamisole activation and there is some evidence that it might augment delayed hypersensitivity reactions. It has been used with good results in the treatment of herpes simplex infections. These features, together with inhibition of growth of some animal tumours, led to its use with cytotoxic agents in a few malignant diseases in man, and further trials are in progress. Though relatively free of serious toxicity, levamisole is not without untoward side effects. Nausea, vomiting, myalgia, rashes and dizziness are among recorded reactions, and a few cases of agranulocytosis have been reported. Levamisole and *C. parvum* are not in general use in cancer chemotherapy.

There are also many other experimental methods by which immune mechanisms are manipulated in an attempt to combat malignant disease. Besides BCG, other mycobacterial fractions have been developed as immunomodulators. Intralymphatic injection of irradiated cellular vaccine has been tried in animals to evoke a greater cellular immune response. Thymosin, a factor from thymus concerned with T cell differentiation and function may have some potential value. Immune RNA is another experimental tool of interest (Pilch et al., 1976). Immune response to transplants can be mediated by immune RNA to cause more rapid rejection of grafts, and this principle has been applied in the treatment of experimental tumours. Preparations of tumours are injected into animals and the resultant immune RNA is extracted from their lymphoid tissues. Another factor, a dialysable component from lysates of leukocytes, can transfer specific cellular immunity from donor to recipient. This activity, attributed to 'transfer factor' was first observed in the transfer of delayed hypersensitivity from donors immune to tuberculin and streptococcal antigen. It has been applied in infections and immune deficiency disorders and there have been a few preliminary studies in malignant disease (LoBuglio and Neidhart, 1976).

Many of these methods depend upon the host's ability to mount the appropriate immune response, whatever that might be. Little as yet is known about such mechanisms, their relation to malignant disease or their interactions with chemotherapy or radiotherapy. As shown in experimental models, immunological intervention can operate adversely and even cause acceleration of tumour growth. Immunotherapy is still considered to be an experimental form of treatment.

Conclusions

Immunotherapy may be classified as active, passive or adoptive. Nonspecific, active immunotherapy with BCG is sometimes used in conjunction with chemotherapy in the treatment of acute leukaemia and other conditions. Several other agents used to stimulate the immune response may have some value in cancer treatment.

Chapter XXVI

Cytotoxic Agents in Non-malignant Conditions

Cytotoxic agents have been tried in a variety of disorders in which pathogenic immune responses occur or are thought to be involved. They are given in an attempt to suppress the reaction or its consequences. Uncontrolled studies make up most of the reports and on the whole the results are disappointing (Gerber and Steinberg, 1976; Skinner and Schwartz, 1972; Skinner and Schwartz, 1972a; Steinberg et al., 1972).

Most experience has centered around cyclophosphamide, azathioprine, mercaptopurine and methotrexate but other drugs such as chlorambucil, vincristine and cytarabine are also used.

Immunosuppression with cytotoxic drugs is usually indicated only when prednisone has proved inadequate or the diseases are severe or rapidly progressive. In many cases the corticosteroid-sparing effect of the cytotoxic drug permits reduction to more tolerable dose levels or, occasionally, the complete suspension of steroids.

In organ transplantation, notably renal transplant, the combination of azathioprine and prednisone is well established for preventing allograft rejection. Worthwhile benefit can be achieved with alkylating agents and the purine antagonists in Wegener's granulomatosis, with more than 60% of patients responding and up to 40% having complete remission of symptoms. Chlorambucil or cyclophosphamide, usually in association with prednisone, are used long term, intermittently, for continuing suppression of the disease. Azathioprine, fluorouracil and methotrexate have also been used with good effect (Fauci et al., 1971). Encouraging results with mithramycin have been reported in Paget's disease of bone.

Some benefit has been observed in cases of dermatomyositis, polymyositis, Reiter's syndrome, psoriasis, pemphigus, chronic ulcerative colitis and chronic active hepatitis. Cyclophosphamide also has a place in selected cases of steroid resistant minimal lesion nephrotic syndrome. The results in idiopathic thrombocytopenic purpura are variable and cytotoxic drugs should be tried only if the response to steroids is poor and splenectomy has failed. Unless the disease presents serious problems, the patient should not be committed to life-long cytotoxic drug therapy (Caplan and Berkman, 1976; Laros and Penner, 1971; Sussman, 1967).

Significant improvement is sometimes seen in cases of severe rheumatoid arthritis, more particularly with high dose cyclophosphamide. The steroid-sparing effect of the alkylating agents has obvious advantages in the long term treatment necessary.

The results of the treatment of systemic lupus erythematosus with cytotoxic drugs are inconsistent, mainly because of the protean nature of the disease and variables in the different reported series. Case selection, different drugs, doses and dose schedules and duration of observation, and incomplete information on the nature of the renal involvement are among the many variables. There are nevertheless a few well documented reports to support the value of azathioprine in diffuse proliferative glomerulonephritis.

Little or no benefit, except perhaps in a few cases, has been seen in scleroderma, Sjogren's syndrome, uveitis, myasthenia gravis, amyloidosis, primary biliary cirrhosis, Goodpasture's disease, Crohn's disease, Guillain Barre syndrome, Behcet's disease and rapidly progressive proliferative glomerulonephritis.

Conclusions

Cytotoxic drugs affect humoral and cell mediated immunity and are used in attempts to suppress pathogenic immune responses. The drugs are well established in preventing allograft rejection. Diseases such as Wegener's granulomatosis, psoriasis and idiopathic thrombocytopenic purpura may respond to cytotoxic drugs.

Chapter XXVII

Present Trends and the Future of Cancer Chemotherapy

The scope of cancer chemotherapy has widened but progress has favoured those diseases shown to respond to the first few drugs developed.

Many thousands of compounds, mostly cytotoxic, have been synthesised or extracted from natural products and screened for anticancer activity, and the search for new drugs continues with optimism. The chemists are not without ingenuity, but their efforts are thwarted by apparent lack of exploitable differences between normal and malignant cells.

Cytotoxic drug therapy seems likely to retain its place in cancer therapeutics for some time yet and there is still a great deal to learn about the optimal use of the available drugs. This includes their earlier application, the revision of current dose schedules and more effective combinations and sequential use of drugs (Cobb, 1970; Cox and Farmer, 1977).

Methods of reducing the morbidity rate are among the most pressing needs of cancer chemotherapy. A morbidity rate is an inevitable consequence of cytotoxic drug treatment in all but the most sensitive of malignant diseases. In relatively resistant disease there is no alternative to the trial of more radical forms of chemotherapy with its attendant toxicity. Regrettably, many patients suffer the side effects without gaining any benefit from treatment. There may be little reason for optimism in these cases, but it is worthwhile remembering that not long ago most children with acute lymphoblastic leukaemia were dying within 6 months of diagnosis and now the median survival time is 3 years.

At the present time, however, it must be admitted that for most of the common forms of malignant disease, chemotherapy has little to offer. In these diseases the drugs are as effective as, 'Eye of newt and toe of frog, Wool of bat and tongue of dog', and a great deal more toxic. The truth remains that cancer chemotherapy needs something completely different.

Appendix

Dose Schedules in Combined Drug Therapy

The details of a few better known combined dose schedules and examples of the type of cancer in which they are used are reproduced here, more for illustration than instruction. Regimens of chemotherapy are often modified in practice, and the literature abounds with variations. Treatment differs with respect to the drugs used, the dose, the duration of administration and the intervals between drugs or cycles, and the number of cycles in each course. The combinations are not necessarily specific for the particular disease for which they were originally prescribed.

MOPP

Mustine	6mg/m^2 IV	day 1 and 8
'Oncovin' (vincristine)	1.4mg/m^2 IV	day 1 and 8
Procarbazine	100mg/m^2 oral	days 1 to 14[1]
Prednisone	40mg/m^2 oral	days 1 to 14[1] (cycles 1 and 4)

6 cycles, at treatment-free intervals of 2 weeks.
Hodgkin's disease.

1 may be given for 10 days only.

MVPP

Mustine	6mg/m^2 IV	day 1 and 8
Vinblastine	6mg/m^2 IV	day 1 and 8
Procarbazine	100mg/m^2 oral	days 1 to 14
Prednisone	40mg/m^2 oral	days 1 to 14

6 cycles, at treatment-free intervals of 28 days.
Hodgkin's disease.

COPP

Cyclophosphamide	450mg/m^2 IV	day 1 and 8
'Oncovin' (vincristine)	1.4mg/m^2 IV	day 1 and 8
Procarbazine	100mg/m^2 oral	days 1 to 10
Prednisone	40mg/m^2 oral	days 1 to 14

6 cycles, at treatment-free intervals of 2 to 3 weeks.
Lymphoma.

COP (or CVP)

[1]Cyclophosphamide	400mg/m^2 oral	days 1 to 5
'Oncovin' (vincristine)	1.4mg/m^2 IV	day 1
Prednisone	60 to 100mg/m^2 oral	days 1 to 5

6 cycles, at treatment-free intervals of 16 days.
Lymphoma.

1 Cyclophosphamide 400 to 800mg/m^2 IV on day 1 may be given instead.

CHOP

Cyclophosphamide	750mg/m^2 IV	day 1
Hydroxydaunorubicin (adriamycin)	50mg/m^2 IV	day 1
'Oncovin' (vincristine)	1.4mg/m^2 IV	day 1
Prednisone	100mg/m^2 oral	days 1 to 5

2 courses, at treatment-free interval of 9 to 16 days.
Lymphomas.

'Seven-three'

Cytarabine	100mg/m^2 IV	days 1 to 7
Daunorubicin	45mg/m^2 IV	days 1 to 3

1 or more courses, at treatment-free intervals of 5 days. May reduce course to 5 and 2 days of cytarabine and daunorubicin respectively.
Acute myeloblastic leukaemia.

COAP

Cyclophosphamide	120mg/m^2 IV	days 1 to 4
'Oncovin' (vincristine)	2mg IV	day 1

Cytarabine	100mg/m^2 IV	days 1 to 4
Prednisone	200mg/m^2 oral	days 1 to 4

1 or more courses, at treatment-free intervals of 14 days.
Acute leukaemia in relapse.

COMB

Cyclophosphamide	1,000mg/m^2 IV	every 6 weeks
'Oncovin' (vincristine)	1mg IV	twice weekly
MethylCCNU (semustine)	100mg/m^2 oral	every 6 weeks
(*or* Methotrexate	50mg oral)	
Bleomycin	30mg IV	twice weekly

Continued if possible until relapse, if responding.
Various carcinomas.

Quadruple Therapy

Vinblastine	6mg/m^2 IV	
Fluorouracil	300mg/m^2 IV	single
Thiotepa	20mg/m^2 IV	administration
Methotrexate	15mg/m^2	

Up to about 24 courses, at treatment-free intervals of 21 to 28 days.
Carcinoma of the breast.

Triple Therapy

CMF

Cyclophosphamide	100mg/m^2 oral	days 1 to 14
Methotrexate	40mg/m^2 IV	day 1 and 8
Fluorouracil	600mg/m^2 IV	day 1 and 8

Courses for 18 months to 2 years, at treatment-free intervals of 2 weeks (or longer).
Carcinoma of the breast.

CMV

Cyclophosphamide	300mg/m^2 IV	
(*or* Thiotepa	20mg/m^2 IV)	single
Methotrexate	60mg/m^2 IV	administration

Vincristine	1.5mg IV
(*or* Vinblastine	10mg IV)

Up to about 24 courses, at treatment free-intervals of 21-28 days.
Carcinoma of the breast.

VAC

Vincristine	1.5mg/m^2 IV	weekly
Actinomycin D	0.6mg/m^2 IV	for
Cyclophosphamide	300mg/m^2 IV	6 weeks

Courses continued, at intervals of 2 weeks for 2 years.
Rhabdomyosarcoma of childhood.

References

Adair, F.E. and Bagg, H.T.: Experimental and clinical studies on the treatment of cancer by dichlorethylsulphide (mustard gas). Annals of Surgery 93: 190-199 (1931).

Aisenberg, A.C. and Goldman, J.M.: Prolongation of survival in Hodgkin's disease. Cancer 27: 802-805 (1970).

Aisner, J.: Platelet transfusion therapy. Medical Clinics of North America 61: 1133-1145 (1977).

Alexanian, R.; Bonnet, J.; Gehan, E.; Haut, A.; Hewlett, J.; Lane, M.; Monto, R. and Wilm, H.: Combination chemotherapy for multiple myeloma. Cancer 30: 382-389 (1972).

Anderson, F.E.; Johnson, A.M. and Havyatt, M.T.: Preliminary studies in the use of 5-fluorouracil cream in the treatment of malignant and premalignant skin tumours. Medical Journal of Australia 2: 385-388 (1969).

Anderson, T. and Young, R.C.: Recent advances in the staging and treatment of ovarian cancer. Medical Clinics of North America 61: 1001-1012 (1977).

Auerbach, C.: Mutagenic effects of alkylating agents. Annals of the New York Academy of Sciences 68: 731-749 (1958).

Bagley, C.M.; Young, R.C.; Canellos, G.P. and DeVita, V.T.: Treatment of ovarian carcinoma: Possibilities for progress. New England Journal of Medicine 287: 856-862 (1972).

Ball, C.R.: Intracellular factors influencing the response of tumours to chemotherapeutic agents. Scientific Basis of Cancer Chemotherapy: Recent Results in Cancer Research Monograph No. 21. Mathe (Ed), p.26-40. Heineman, London (1969).

Belisario, J.C.: Topical cytotoxic therapy of solar keratoses with 5-fluorouracil. Medical Journal of Australia 2: 1136-1140 (1969).

Bender, R.A. and Dedrick, R.L.: Cytokinetic aspects of clinical drug resistance. Cancer Chemotherapy Reports 59: 805-809 (1975).

Benjamin, R.S.; Baker, L.H.; O'Bryan, R.M.; Moon, T.E. and Gottlieb, J.A.: Advances in the chemotherapy of soft tissue sarcomas. Medical Clinics of North America 61: 1039-1043 (1977).

Berenbaum, M.C.: The last surviving cancer cell: The chances of killing it. Cancer Chemotherapy Reports 52: 539-541 (1968).

Bernard, J. and Boiron, M.: Current status: Treatment of acute leukaemia. Seminars in Haematology 7: 427-440 (1970).

Bloom, H.J.G. and Wallace, D.M.: Hormones and the kidney: Possible therapeutic role of testosterone in a patient with regression of metastases from renal adenocarcinoma. British Medical Journal 3: 476-480 (1964).

Bonadonna, G. and Monfardini, S.: Chemotherapy of non-Hodgkin's lymphomas. Cancer Treatment Reviews 1: 167-181 (1974).

Bonadonna, G.; Brusamolino, E.; Valagussa, P.; Rossi, A.; DeLena, M.; Tancini, G.; Bajetta, E.; Musumeci, R. and Veronesi, U.: Combination chemotherapy as an adjunct treatment in operable breast cancer. New England Journal of Medicine 294: 405-410 (1976).

Bonadonna, G.; Zuceli, R.; DeLena, M. and Valagussa, P.: Combined chemotherapy (MOPP or ABVD)-radiotherapy approach in advanced Hodgkin's disease. Cancer Treatment Reports 61: 769-777 (1977).

Broder, C.E. and Carbone, P.P.: Pharmacokinetic considerations in the design of optimal chemotherapeutic regimens for the treatment of breast carcinoma. A conceptual approach. Medical and Pediatric Oncology 2: 11-27 (1976).

Bruce, W.R.; Meeker, B.E. and Valeriote, F.A.: Comparison of the similarity of normal haematopoietic and transplanted lymphoma colony-forming cells to chemotherapeutic agents administered in vivo. Journal of the National Cancer Institute 37: 233-245 (1966).

Buchler, D.A.; Kline, J.C.; Davis, H.; Ramerez, G. and Carr, W.: Treatment and results: Stage III ovarian carcinoma. 11th International Cancer Congress Abstracts, 565-566 (1974).

Bull, C.A.; Biggs, J.C.; Newton, N.C.; de Wilde, F.W. and Chew, K.M.: Bleomycin in squamous cell carcinoma. Medical Journal of Australia 2: 704-707 (1972).

Bunn, P.A.: Should ineffective agents be used in combination chemotherapy. Cancer Chemotherapy Reports 58: 127-128 (1974).

Bunn, P.A.; Cohen, M.H.; Ihde, D.C.; Fossieck, B.E.; Matthews, M.J. and Minna, J.D.: Advances in small cell bronchogenic cancer. Cancer Treatment Reports 61: 733-742 (1977).

Burchenal, J.H. and Carter, S.K.: New cancer chemotherapeutic agents. Cancer 30: 1639-1646 (1972).

Burchenal, J.H.; Murphy, M.I.; Ellison, R.R.; Sykes, M.P.; Tan, T.C.; Leone, I.A.; Karnofsky, D.A.; Craver, L.F.; Dargeon, H.W. and Rhoads, C.P.: Clinical evaluation of a new antimetabolite, 6-mercaptopurine in the treatment of leukaemia and allied diseases. Blood 8: 965-999 (1953).

Burchenal, J.H. and Karnofsky, D.A.: Clinical evaluation of L-asparaginase. Cancer 25: 241-243 (1970).

Cady, B.: Current philosophy in treatment of primary cancer of the breast. Medical Clinics of North America 59: 285-292 (1975).

Cady, B.: Chemotherapy concepts in malignant melanoma. Medical Clinics of North America 59: 305-308 (1975a).

Caplan, S.N. and Berkman, E.M.: Immunosuppressive therapy of idiopathic thrombocytopenia. Medical Clinics of North America 60: 971-986 (1976).

Canellos, G.P.: Chronic granulocytic leukaemia. Medical Clinics of North America 60: 1001-1018 (1976).

Carbone, P.P.; Bono, V.; Frei, E. and Brindley, C.O.: Clinical studies with vincristine. Blood 21: 640-647 (1963).

Carbone, P.P.: Non-Hodgkin's lymphoma: Recent observations on natural history and intensive treatment. Cancer 30: 1511-1516 (1972).

Carter, S.K.: An overview of the status of the nitrosoureas in other tumours. Cancer Chemotherapy Reports 4: Part 3 No. 3 35-46 (1973).

Carter, S.K. and Soper, W.T.: Integration of chemotherapy into combined modality treatment of solid tumours: I. The overall strategy. Cancer Treatment Reviews 1: 1-13 (1974).

Carter, S.K. and Livingston, R.B.: Cyclophosphamide in solid tumours. Cancer Treatment Reviews 2: 295-322 (1975).

Carter, S.K.: Integration of chemotherapy into combined modality treatment of solid tumours. VII Adenocarcinoma of breast. Cancer Treatment Reviews 3: 141-174 (1976).

Chang, P.: Progress in the treatment of osteosarcoma. Medical Clinics of North America 61: 1027-1038 (1977).

Clifford, P.; Singh, S.; Stjersward, J. and Klein, G.: Long term survival of patients with Burkitt's lymphoma: An assessment of treatment and other factors which may relate to survival. Cancer Research 27: 2578-2615 (1967).

Cobb, L.M.: Tissue specific chemotherapy. Cancer Chemotherapy Reports 54: 375-378 (1970).

Cohen, F.B.; Lippman, A.J.; Custodio, M.C. and Decter, J.A.: New antineoplastic drugs and their proper use. Medical Clinics of North America 60: 959-970 (1976).

Cohlan, S.Q.: The teratogenicity of drugs in man. Pharmacology for Physicians 3: 1-5 (1969).

Condit, P.T.: Chemotherapy of neoplastic disease with folate antagonists. Annals of the New York Academy of Sciences 186: 475-485 (1971).

Costa, G.; Engle, R.L.; Schilling, A.; Carbone, P.; Kochwa, S.; Nachman, R.L. and Glidewell, O.: Melphalan and prednisone: An effective combination for the treatment of multiple myeloma. American Journal of Medicine 54: 589-599 (1973).

Cox, P.J. and Farmer, P.B.: Towards selectivity? Approaches to the design of new anticancer agents. Cancer Treatment Reviews 4: 48-63 (1977).

Cridland, M.D.: Antineoplastic and immunosuppressive drugs: III: Adverse effects and therapeutic problems. Drugs 3: 352-365 (1972).

Cridland, M.D.: Chronic lymphocytic leukaemia. Medical Journal of Australia 2: 17-19 (1974).

Cridland, M.D. and Green, D.: The management of generalised lymphosarcomatous disease. Medical Journal of Australia 2: 195-201 (1968).

Crivelli, G.; Monfardini, S.; Morello, G. and Bonadonna, G.: Radiation therapy, BCNU and CCNU in the treatment of malignant glioma. 11th International Cancer Congress Abstracts 574-575 (1974).

Crowther, D.; Bateman, C.J.T.; Vartan, C.P.; Whitehouse, J.M.A.; Malpas, J.S.; Fairley, G.H. and Scott, R.B.: Combination chemotherapy using l-asparaginase, daunorubicin and cytosine arabinoside in adults with acute myelogenous leukaemia. British Medical Journal 4: 513-517 (1970).

Crowther, D.; Powles, R.L.; Bateman, C.J.T.; Malpas, J.S.: Fairley, G.H. and Scott, R.B.: Management of adult acute myelogenous leukaemia. British Medical Journal 1: 131-137 (1973).

Dameshek, W.: Comments on the therapy of polycythemia vera. Seminars in Haematology 3: 226-227 (1966).

Dameshek, W.; Granville, N.B. and Rubio, F.: Therapy of the myeloproliferative disorders with Myleran. Annals of the New York Academy of Sciences 68: 1001-1006 (1958).

Desai, D.V.; Ezdinli, E.Z. and Stutzman, L.: Vincristine therapy of lymphomas and chronic lymphocytic leukaemia. Cancer 26: 352-359 (1970).

De Vita, V.T.; Serpick, A.A. and Carbone, P.P.: Combination chemotherapy in the treatment of advanced Hodgkin's disease. Annals of Internal Medicine 73: 881-1035 (1970).

De Vita, V.T.; Canellos, G.P. and Moxley, J.H.: A decade of combination chemotherapy of advanced Hodgkin's disease. Cancer 30: 1495-1504 (1972).

De Vita, V.T. and Carbone, P.P.: Chemotherapeutic implications of staging in Hodgkin's disease. Cancer Research 31: 1838-1844 (1971).

De Vita, V.T. and Schein, P.S.: The use of drugs in combination for the treatment of cancer: Rationale and Results. New England Journal of Medicine 288: 998-1006 (1973).

Di Paolo, J.A.: Teratogenic Agents: Mammalian test systems and chemicals. Annals of the New York Academy of Sciences 163: 801-812 (1969).

Donaldson, S.S.; Castro, J.R.; Wilbur, J.R. and Jesse, R.H.: Rhabdomyosarcoma of head and neck in children. Combination treatment by surgery, irradiation and chemotherapy. Cancer 31: 26-35 (1973).

Donovan, J.E.: Non-hormonal chemotherapy of adenocarcinoma of the uterus. A review. 11th International Cancer Congress Abstracts, 564-565 (1974).

Douglas, I.D.C. and Price, L.A.: Bone marrow toxicity of methotrexate: A reassessment. British Journal of Haematology 24: 625-631 (1973).

Editorial: Asparaginase. Medical Journal of Australia 2: 1045-1046 (1971).

Elson, L.A.: Haematological effects of the alkylating agents. Annals of the New York Academy of Sciences 68: 826-833 (1958).

Epstein, E.H.; Levin, D.L.; Croft, J.D. and Lutzner, M.A.: Mycosis fungoides. Survival, prognostic features, response to therapy and autopsy findings. Medicine 15: 61-72 (1972).

Evans, A.E.; Heyn, R.M.; Newton, W.A. and Leiken, S.L.: Vincristine sulphate and cyclophosphamide for children with metastatic neuroblastoma. Journal of the American Medical Association 207: 1325-1327 (1969).

Ezdinli, E.Z. and Stutzman, L.: Chlorambucil therapy for lymphomas and chronic lymphocytic leukaemia. Journal of the American Medical Association 191: 444-450 (1965).

Farber, S.: Chemotherapy in the treatment of leukaemia and Wilm's tumour. Journal of the American Medical Association 198: 154-164 (1966).

Farber, S.; Diamond, L.K.; Mercer, R.D.; Sylvester, R.F. and Wolff, J.A.: Temporary remissions in acute leukaemia in children produced by folic acid antagonists, 4-aminopteroyl-glutamic acid (aminopterin). New England Journal of Medicine 238: 787-793 (1948).

Fauci, A.S.; Wolff, S.M. and Johnson, J.S.: Effect of cyclophosphamide upon the immune response in Wegener's granulomatosis. New England Journal of Medicine 285: 1493-1496 (1971).

Fernbach, D.J.; Sutow, W.W.; Thurman, W.G. and Vietti, T.J.: Preliminary clinical trials with cyclophosphamide in children with acute leukaemia. Cancer Chemotherapy Reports 8: 102-105 (1960).

Fisher, B.: Adjuvant chemotherapy in the primary management of breast cancer. Medical Clinics of North America 61: 953-965 (1977).

Fisher, B.; Carbone, P.; Economou, S.G.; Frielich, R.; Glass, A.; Lerner, H.; Redmond, C.; Zelen, M.; Band, P.; Katrych, D.; Wolmark, N. and Fisher, E.: L-phenylalanine mustard (1-PAM) in the management of primary breast cancer. A report of early findings. New England Journal of Medicine 292: 117-122 (1975).

Frei, E.: Prospectus for cancer chemotherapy. Cancer 30: 1656-1661 (1972).

Frei, E. and Gehan, E.A.: Definition of cure for Hodgkin's disease. Cancer Research 31: 1828-1833 (1971).

Freireich, D.J.; Karon, M. and Frei, E.: Quadruple combination chemotherapy (VAMP) for acute lymphocytic leukaemia of childhood. Proceedings of the American Association for Cancer Research 5: 20 (1964).

Friedman, M.; Nervi, C.; Casale, C.; Starace, G.; Arcangeli, G.; Page, G. and Ziparo, E.: Significance of growth rates, cell kinetics, and histology in the irradiation and chemotherapy of squamous cell carcinoma of the mouth. Cancer 31: 10-16 (1972).

Galton, D.A.G.: Myleran in chronic myeloid leukaemia. Lancet 1: 208-213 (1953).

Galton, D.A.G.: The treatment of chronic leukaemias. British Medical Bulletin 15: 78-85 (1959).

Galton, D.A.G.: Chemotherapy of chronic myelocytic leukaemia. Seminars in Haematology 6: 323-343 (1969).

Galton, D.A.G.; Till, M. and Wiltshaw, E.: Busulphan (1,4-di-methane-sulphonyloxybutane, Myleran): Summary of clinical results. Annals of the New York Academy of Sciences 68: 967-973 (1958).

Gamble, J.F.; Fuller, L.M.; Ibrahim, E. et al.: Combined chemotherapy radiotherapy management of stage III Hodgkin's disease. Archives of Internal Medicine 131: 435-438 (1973).

George, R.P.: Poth, J.I.; Gordon, D. and Schrier, S.I.: Multiple myeloma — intermittent combination chemotherapy compared to continuous therapy. Cancer 29: 1665-1670 (1971).

Gerber, N.L. and Steinberg, A.D.: Clinical use of immunosuppressive drugs: Part II. Drugs 11: 90-112 (1976).

Goldie, J.H.; Price, L.A. and Harrap, K.R.: Methotrexate toxicity: Correlation with duration of administration, plasma levels, dose and excretion pattern. European Journal of Cancer 6: 409-411 (1972).

Goldin, A.: Combination chemotherapy with folate antagonists. Annals of the New York Academy of Sciences 186: 423-437 (1971).

Goodman, L.S.; Wintrobe, M.M.; Dameshek, W.; Goodman, M.J.; Gelman, A. and McLennan, M.T.: Nitrogen mustard therapy. Journal of the American Medical Association 132: 126-132 (1946).

Gottlieb, J.A. and Drewinko, B.: Review of current clinical status of platinum coordination complexes in cancer chemotherapy. Cancer Chemotherapy Reports 59: 621-628 (1975).

Gray, P. and Michaels, L.: Bleomycin in advanced squamous cell carcinoma of head and neck. Medical Journal of Australia 2: 246-249 (1972).

Gunz, F.W. and Vincent, P.C.: Towards a cure of acute granulocytic leukaemia? Leukaemia Research 1: 51-66 (1977).

Gutterman, J.U.; Mavligit, G.M. and Hersh, E.M.: Chemotherapy of human solid tumours. Medical Clinics of North America 60: 441-462 (1976).

Haddow, A.: Mechanisms of carcinogenesis. II Biological alkylating agents: in Homburger and Fishman (Eds) The Physiopathology of Cancer, p.478 (Hoeber, New York 1953).

Haddow, A. and Timmis, G.M.: Myleran in chronic myeloid leukaemia. Chemical constitution and biological action. Lancet 1: 207 (1953).

Halnan, K.E.; Bleehen, N.M.; Brewin, T.B.; Deeley, T.J.; Harrison, D.F.N.; Howland, C.; Kunkler, P.B.; Ritchie, G.L.; Wiltshaw, E. and Todd, I.D.H.: Early clinical experience with bleomycin in the United Kingdom in series of 105 patients. British Medical Journal 4: 635-638 (1972).

Hammond, C.B. and Parker, R.T.: Diagnosis and treatment of trophoblastic disease. Journal of Obstetrics and Gynaecology 35: 132-143 (1970).

Hansen, H.H.: Management of lung cancer. Medical Clinics of North America 61: 979-989 (1977).

Harrap, K.R.; Hill, B.T.; Furness, M.E. and Hart, L.I.: Sites of action of amethopterin: Intrinsic and acquired drug resistance. Annals of the New York Academy of Sciences 186: 312-324 (1971).

Haskell, C.M.: Management of metastatic breast cancer. Medical Clinics of North America 61: 967-978 (1977).

Heal, J.M. and Schein, P.S.: Management of gastrointestinal cancer. Medical Clinics of North America 61: 991-999 (1977).

Hemsworth, B.N. and Jackson, H.: Embryopathies induced by cytotoxic substances; in Robson, Sullivan and Smith (Eds) A Symposium on Embryopathic Activity of Drugs p.116-137 (Churchill, London 1965).

Henderson, E.S.: Combination chemotherapy of acute lymphocytic leukaemia of childhood. Cancer Research 27: 2570-2572 (1967).

Henderson, E.S.: Treatment of acute leukaemia. Seminars in Haematology 6: 271-319 (1969).

Hersh, E.M.; Gutterman, J.U. and Mavligit, G.M.: Immunotherapy of leukaemia. Medical Clinics of North America 60: 1019-1042 (1976).

Herz, R.; Ross, G.T. and Lipsett, M.B.: Chemotherapy in women with trophoblastic disease. Wisconsin Medical Journal 64: 190-193 (1965).

Heyn, R.; Borges, W.; Joo, P.; Karon, M.; Nesbit, M.; Shore, N.; Breslow, N. and Hammond, D.: BCG in the treatment of acute lymphocytic leukaemia (ALL). Proceedings of the American Association for Cancer Research 14: 45 (1973).

Hill, A.B.: Clinical trials; in Principles of Medical Statistics p.243-266 (The Lancet Ltd. London 1967).

Hill, B.T. and Baserga, R.: The cell cycle and its significance for cancer treatment. Cancer Treatment Reviews 2: 159-175 (1975).

Hill, J.M.; Loeb, E.; MacLellan, A.M.; Hill, N.O.; Khan, A. and King, J.J.: Clinical studies of platinum coordination compounds in the treatment of various malignant diseases. Cancer Chemotherapy Reports 59: 647-659 (1975).

Hill, J.M. and Loeb, E.: Treatment of leukaemia, lymphoma and other malignant neoplasms with vinblastine. Cancer Chemotherapy Reports 15: 41-61 (1961).

Hodes, M.E.; Rohn, R.J. and Bond, W.H.: Vincaleukoblastine: I. Preliminary clinical studies. Cancer Research 20: 1041-1049 (1960).

Hodes, M.E.; Rohn, R.J.; Bond, W.H.; Yardley, J.M. and Corpening, W.S.: Vincaleukoblastine. IV Summary of 2 and one half years' experience in use of vinblastine. Cancer Chemotherapy Reports 16: 401-406 (1962).

Holland, J.F.: Chemotherapeutic goals in acute leukaemia. New England Journal of Medicine 280: 216-217 (1969).

Holland, J.F. and Glidewell, O.: Chemotherapy of acute lymphocytic leukaemia of childhood. Cancer 30: 1480-1487 (1972).

Holoye, P.Y. and Samuels, M.: Bleomycin-Velban combination in metastatic testicular neoplasms. 11th International Cancer Congress Abstracts, 857-858 (1974).

Hoogstraten, B.; Holland, J.F.; Kramer, S. and Glidewell, O.J.: Combination chemotherapy-radiotherapy for stage III Hodgkin's disease. Archives of Internal Medicine 131: 424-428 (1973).

Hryniuk, W.M. and Bertino, J.R.: Growth rate and cell kill. Annals of the New York Academy of Sciences 186: 330-342 (1971).

Humphreys, S.R. and Karrer, K.: Relationship of dose schedules to the effectiveness of adjuvant chemotherapy. Cancer Chemotherapy Reports 54: 379-392 (1970).

Irvine, W.T. and Luck, R.J.: Review of regional limb perfusion with melphalan for malignant melanoma. British Medical Journal 1: 770-774 (1966).

Jacquillat, C.; Weil, M.; Gemon, M.F.; Izrael, V.; Schaison, G.; Auclerc, G.; Ablin, A.R.; Flandrin, G.; Tanzer, J.; Bussel, A.; Weisgerber, C.; Dresch, C.; Najean, Y.; Goudemand, M.; Seligmann, M.; Boiron, M. and Bernard, J.: Evaluation of 216 four-year survivors of acute leukaemia. Cancer 32: 286-293 (1973).

Jaffe, N.: Progress on high dose methotrexate (NSC-740) with citrovorum rescue in the treatment of metastatic bone tumours. Cancer Chemotherapy Reports 58: 275-280 (1974).

Jaffe, N.: Treatment of bone tumours: Chemotherapy (methods and results). 11th International Cancer Congress Abstracts 101-102 (1974a).

Jeliffe, A.M.: Value of prednisone in combination chemotherapy of stage IV Hodgkin's disease. British Medical Journal 3: 413-415 (1975).

Johnson, I.S.; Wright, H.K.; Svoboda, G.H. and Vlantis, J.: Antitumour principles derived from Vinca rosea Linn. I. Vincaleukoblastine and Leurosine. Cancer Research 20: 1016-1022 (1960).

Johnson, R.E.: Modern approaches to the radiotherapy of lymphomas. Seminars in Haematology 6: 357-375 (1969).

Johnson, R.E.; O-Conor, G.T. and Levin, D.: Primary management of advanced lymphosarcoma with radiotherapy. Cancer 25: 787-791 (1970a).

Johnson, R.E.; Thomas, L.B.; Schneiderman, M.; Glenn, D.W.; Faw, F. and Hafermann, M.D.: Preliminary experience with total nodal irradiation in Hodgkin's disease. Radiology 96: 603-608 (1970).

Johnson, R.E.; Glover, M.K. and Marshall, S.K.: Results of radiation therapy and implications for the clinical staging of Hodgkin's disease. Cancer Research 31: 1834-1837 (1971).

Johnson, R.E.: Remission induction and remission duration with primary radiotherapy in advanced lymphosarcoma. Cancer 29: 1473-1476 (1972).

Johnson, C.E.; Decker, D.G.; Van Herick, M. and Nussey, E.: Advanced ovarian cancer: Therapy with radiation and cyclophosphamide in a random series. American Journal of Roentgenology 114: 136-141 (1972).

Kaplan, H.S.: Role of intensive radiotherapy in the management of Hodgkin's disease. Cancer 19: 358-367 (1966).

Kaplan, H.S.: Clinical evaluation and radiotherapeutic management of Hodgkin's disease and the malignant lymphomas. New England Journal of Medicine 278: 892-899 (1968).

Karnofsky, D.A.: Summary of results obtained with nitrogen mustard in the treatment of neoplastic disease. Annals of the New York Academy of Sciences 68: 899-914 (1958).

Kaung, D.T.; Close, H.P.; Whittington, R.M. and Patno, M.E.: Comparison of busulphan and cyclophosphamide in the treatment of chronic myelocytic leukaemia. Cancer 27: 608-612 (1971).

Kennedy, B.J.: Mithramycin therapy of advanced testis cancer. 11th International Cancer Congress Abstracts 856-857 (1974).

Kennedy, B.J. and Yarbro, T.W.: Metabolic and therapeutic effects of hydroxyurea in chronic myeloid leukaemia. Journal of the American Medical Association 195: 1038-1043 (1966).

Killmann, S.A.: Kinetics of leukaemic blast cells in man. Clinics in Haematology 1: 95-113 (1972).

Krementz, E.T.; Ryan, R.F.; Carter, R.D. and Sutherland, C.M.: Chemotherapy by perfusion for melanoma of the limbs. 11th International Cancer Congress Abstracts 538-539 (1974).

Kuhbock, J.; Gruber, F.; Klicpera, M.; Miraghai, J.; Potzi, P. and Weidinger, P.: Therapeutic results and side effects of mithramycin in the treatment of testicular tumours. 11th International Cancer Congress Abstracts 857 (1974).

Lacher, M.J. and Durant, J.R.: Combined vinblastine and chlorambucil therapy of Hodgkin's disease. Annals of Internal Medicine 62: 468-476 (1963).

Laros, R.K. and Penner, J.A.: 'Refractory' thrombocytopenic purpura treated successfully with cyclophosphamide. Journal of the American Medical Association 215: 445-449 (1971).

Leading Article: Chemotherapy in breast cancer. British Medical Journal 2: 832 (1976).

Lee, Y.T.N. and Spratt, J.S.: Malignant Lymphoma. Nodal and Extranodal Diseases. Modern Surgical Monographs. Grune and Stratton, New York (1974).

Lenaz, L. and Page, J.A.: Cardiotoxicity of adriamycin and related anthracyclines. Cancer Treatment Reviews 3: 111-120 (1976).

Lichtenfield, J.L.: Malignant melanoma. Medical Clinics of North America 61: 1013-1025 (1977).

LoBuglio, A.F. and Neidhart, J.A.: Transfer factor. A potential agent for cancer therapy. Medical Clinics of North America 60: 585-590 (1976).

Luce, J.K.; Frei, E.; Gehan, E.A.; Coltman, C.A.; Talley, R. and Monto, R.W.: Chemotherapy of Hodgkin's disease. Maintenance therapy vs. no maintenance therapy after remission induction with combination chemotherapy. Archives of Internal Medicine 131: 391-395 (1973).

McElwain, T.J.; Atkinson, K. and Peckham, M.J.: Chemotherapy for testicular teratoma. 11th International Cancer Congress Abstracts 858 (1974).

McKneally, M.F.; Maver, C. and Kausel, H.W.: Regional immunotherapy of lung cancer with intrapleural BCG. Lancet 1: 377-379 (1976).

Malkasian, G.D.: Chemotherapy for ovarian cancer. Medical Clinics of North America 58: 779-792 (1974).

Malling, H.V. and de Serres, F.J.: Mutagenicity of alkylating carcinogens. Annals of the New York Academy of Sciences 163: 788-800 (1969).

Malpas, J.J.; Freeman, J.E.; Paxton, A. and Wood, C.B.S.: The treatment of rhabdomyosarcoma in children. 11th International Cancer Congress Abstracts, 795 (1974).

Mansfield, C.M.: Early Breast Cancer. Its History and Results of Treatment. Experimental Biology and Medicine Monograph No. 5. Wolsky (Ed) Karger, Basel (1976).

Marmont, A.M. and Damasio, E.E.: The effects of two alkaloids derived from Vinca rosea on the malignant cells of Hodgkin's disease, lymphosarcoma and acute leukaemia in vivo. Blood 29: 1-21 (1967).

Mathe, G.: Operational Research in Cancer Chemotherapy. Chemotherapy in the Strategy of Cancer Treatment; in Scientific Basis of Cancer Chemotherapy: Recent Results in Cancer Research (Monograph No. 21), p.72-96 Mathe (Ed). Heinemann, London (1969).

Mathe, G.: Advances in the treatment of acute (blastic) leukaemias: Recent Results in Cancer Research, Volume 30. Mathe (Ed). Heinemann, London (1970).

Mathe, G.; Redon, H. and Hyet, M.: Study of the clinical efficiency of bleomycin in human cancer. British Medical Journal 2: 643-645 (1970).

Medical Research Council: Chronic granulocytic leukaemia: Comparison of radiotherapy and busulphan therapy. British Medical Journal 1: 201-208 (1968).

Medical Research Council: Treatment of acute lymphoblastic leukaemia. Comparison of immunotherapy (BCG), intermittent methotrexate and no therapy after a five-month intensive cytotoxic regimen. British Medical Journal 4: 189-194 (1971).

Miller, D.G.: Alkylating agents and human spermatogenesis. Journal of the American Medical Association 217: 162-1665 (1971).

Moertel, C.G.: Chemotherapy of upper gastrointestinal carcinoma. British Journal of Cancer 34: 325-334 (1976).

Morton, D.C.; Eilber, F.R.; Holmes, E.C.; Sparks, F.C. and Ramming, K.: BCG immunotherapy as a systemic adjunct to surgery in malignant melanoma. Medical Clinics of North America 60: 431-439 (1976).

Murphy, M.L.; DelMoro, G. and Lacon, C.: The comparative effects of five polyfunctional alkylating agents on the rat fetus, with additional notes on the chick embryo. Annals of the New York Academy of Sciences 68: 762-782 (1958).

Nicholson, W.M.; Beard, M.E.J.; Crowther, D.; Stansfield, A.G.; Vartan, C.P.; Malpas, J.S.; Fairley, G.H. and Scott, R.B.: Combination chemotherapy in generalised Hodgkin's disease. British Medical Journal 3: 7-10 (1970).

Nissen, N.I.; Stutzman, L.; Holland, J.F. and Glidewell, O.J.: Chemotherapy of Hodgkin's disease in studies by Acute Leukaemia Group B. Archives of Internal Medicine 131: 395-401 (1973).

Oberfield, R.A.: Current status of regional arterial infusion chemotherapy. Medical Clinics of North America 59: 411-424 (1975).

Ochoa, M.; Alkylating agents in clinical cancer chemotherapy. Annals of the New York Academy of Sciences 163: 921-930 (1969).

Oettgen, H.F.; Pinsky, C.M. and Delmonte, L.: Treatment of cancer with immunomodulators Corynecbacterium parvum and levamisole. Medical Clinics of North America 60: 511-537 (1976).

Oliverio, V.T. and Zaharko, D.S.: Tissue distribution of folate antagonists. Annals of the New York Academy of Sciences 186: 387-399 (1971).

O'Loughlin, J.M.: Infections in the immunosuppressed patient. Medical Clinics of North America 59: 495-501 (1975).

Perry, S.; Thomas, L.B.; Johnson, R.E.; Carbone, P.P. and Haynes, H.A.: Hodgkin's disease. Annals of Internal Medicine 67: 424-442 (1967).

Peters, M.V.; Alison, R.E. and Bush, R.S.: Natural history of Hodgkin's disease as related to staging. Cancer 19: 308-316 (1966).

Pilch, Y.H.; Fritze, D. and Kern, D.H.: Immune RNA in the immunotherapy of cancer. Medical Clinics of North America 60: 567-583 (1976).

Powell, H.R. and Ekert, H.: Methotrexate induced congenital malformations. Medical Journal of Australia 2: 1076-1077 (1971).

Powles, R.L.: Immunologic maneuvers in the management of acute leukaemia. Medical Clinics of North America 60: 463-472 (1976).

Price, C.C.: Fundamental mechanisms of alkylation. Annals of the New York Academy of Sciences 68: 663-668 (1958).

Price, C.C.; Gaucher, G.M.; Koneru, P.; Shibakawa, R.; Sowa, J.R. and Yamaguchi, M.: Mechanism of action of alkylating agents. Annals of the New York Academy of Sciences 163: 593-600 (1969).

Rapoport, A.; Cole, P. and Mason, J.: Correlates of survival after initiation of chemotherapy in 142 cases of Hodgkin's disease. Cancer 23: 377-381 (1969).

Reimer, R.R.; Hoover, R.; Fraumeni, J.F. and Young, R.C.: Acute leukaemia after alkylating agent therapy of ovarian cancer. New England Journal of Medicine 297: 177-181 (1977).

Rhoads, C.P.: Nitrogen mustards in treatment of neoplastic disease: Official statement. Journal of the American Medical Association 131: 656-658 (1946).

Richter, P.; Calamera, J.C.; Morgenfeld, M.C.; Kierszenbaum, A.L.; Lavieri, J.C. and Mancini, R.E.: Effect of chlorambucil on spermatogenesis in the human with malignant lymphoma. Cancer 25: 1026-1030 (1960).

Rivers, S.L. and Patno, M.E.: Cyclophosphamide vs. melphalan in treatment of plasma cell myeloma. Journal of the American Medical Association 207: 1328-1334 (1969).

Rosen, B.J.: Multiple myeloma. A clinical review. Medical Clinics of North America 59: 375-386 (1975).

Rosenberg, B.: Possible mechanisms for the antitumour activity of platinum coordination complexes. Cancer Chemotherapy Reports 59: 589-598 (1975).

Rosenoer, V.M. and Curby, W.A.: Growth kinetics of solid tumours: Implications for chemotherapy. Medical Clinics of North America 59: 339-346 (1975).

Rubens, R.D.; Wiltshaw, E.; Boesen, E. and Galton, D.A.G.: Multiple drug therapy in Hodgkin's disease. European Journal of Cancer 8: 477-484 (1972).

Sahakian, G.J.: Management of Hodgkin's and non-Hodgkin's lymphomas. Medical Clinics of North America 59: 387-397 (1975).

Schajowicz, D.F.; Estevez, R. and Chacon, R.: Treatment of Ewing's sarcoma. 11th International Cancer Congress Abstracts, 794-795 (1974).

Schiffer, C.A.: Principles of granulocyte transfusion therapy. Medical Clinics of North America 61: 1119-1131 (1977).

Schimpff, S.C.: Therapy of infection in patients with granulocytopenia. Medical Clinics of North America 61: 1101-1118 (1977).

Schwartz, A.D.: Neuroblastoma and Wilms' tumour. Medical Clinics of North America 61: 1053-1071 (1977).

Schwartz, P.E. and Smith, J.F.: Treatment of ovarian stromal tumours. American Journal of Obstetrics and Gynecology 125: 402-411 (1976).

Scott, H.; Stephenson, R.T.; Fox, W. and Roy, D.L.: 6 year follow-up of cytotoxic chemotherapy as an adjunct to surgery in carcinoma of the bronchus. British Journal of Cancer 34: 167-173 (1976).

Shapiro, W.R.: Chemotherapy of malignant glioma with BCNU, vincristine sulphate and CCNU. 11th International Cancer Congress Abstracts, 575-576 (1974).

Silver, R.T.: The treatment of chronic lymphocytic leukaemia. Seminars in Haematology 6: 344-356 (1969).

Simone, J.; Aur, R.J.A.; Hustu, H.O. and Pinkel, D.: 'Total therapy' studies of acute lymphocytic leukaemia in children. Current results and prospects for cure. Cancer 30: 1488-1494 (1972).

Skinner, M.D. and Schwartz, R.S.: Immunosuppressive therapy. New England Journal of Medicine 287: 221-226 (1972).

Skinner, M.D. and Schwartz, R.S.: Immunosuppressive therapy. New England Journal of Medicine 287: 281-286 (1972a).

Skipper, H.E.; Schabel, F.M. and Wilcox, W.S.: Experimental evaluation of potential anticancer agents. XIII. On the criteria and kinetics associated with 'curability' of experimental leukaemia. Cancer Chemotherapy Reports 35: 1-111 (1964).

Skipper, H.E.; Schabel, F.M. and Wilcox, W.S.: Experimental evaluation of potential anticancer agents. XIV. Further study of certain basic concepts underlying chemotherapy of leukaemia. Cancer Chemotherapy Reports 45: 5-28 (1965).

Skipper, H.E.: Combination chemotherapy. Some concepts and results. Cancer Chemotherapy Reports 4: 137-145 (1974).

Sparks, F.C.: Hazards and complications of BCG immunotherapy. Medical Clinics of North America 60: 499-509 (1976).

Sparks, F.C.; Silverstein, M.J.; Hunt, J.S.; Haskell, C.M.; Pilch, Y.H. and Morton, D.L.: Complications of BCG immunotherapy in patients with cancer. New England Journal of Medicine 289: 827-830 (1973).

Spiers, A.S.D.: Experience with procarbazine in the treatment of acute leukaemia and other neoplasms. Medical Journal of Australia 2: 732-735 (1967).

Smith, P.K.; Madkarni, M.V.; Trams, E.G. and Davidson, C.: Distribution and fate of alkylating agents. Annals of the New York Academy of Sciences 68: 834-852 (1958).

Steinberg, D.: The management of acute myelogenous leukaemia. Medical Clinics of North America 59: 363-373 (1975).

Steinberg, A.D.; Plotz, P.H.; Wolff, S.M.; Wong, V.G.; Agus, S.G. and Decker, J.L.: Cytotoxic drugs in treatment of nonmalignant diseases. Annals of Internal Medicine 76: 619-642 (1972).

Steinberg, S.S.; Philips, F.S. and Scholler, J.: Pharmacological and pathological effects of alkylating agents. Annals of the New York Academy of Sciences 68: 811-825 (1958).

Stewart, G.R.: Intraarterial infusion of cytotoxic agents. Medical Journal of Australia 1: 300-305 (1970).

Storring, R.A.; Jameson, B.; McElwain, T.J.; Wiltshaw, E.; Spiers, A.S.D. and Gaya, H.: Oral non-absorbable antibiotics prevent infection in acute non-lymphoblastic leukaemia. Lancet 2: 837-840 (1977).

Stutzman, L.: Combined radiotherapy and chemotherapy of lymphomas and other cancers. Cancer Research 31: 1845-1850 (1971).

Sturtz, A.J.; Greenberg, A.J.; Wiley, A.; Gilbert, E.F. and Oppenheimer, J.: Burkitt's lymphoma: The role of radiotherapy. Radiology 104: 379-384 (1972).

Sussman, L.N.: Azathioprine in refractory idiopathic thrombocytopenic purpura. Journal of the American Medical Association 202: 259-263 (1967).

Tattersall, M.H.N. and Harrap, K.R.: Combination chemotherapy: The antagonism of methotrexate and cytosine arabinoside. European Journal of Cancer 9: 229-232 (1973).

Tattersall, M.H.N.; Jackson, R.C.; Connors, T.A. and Harrap, K.R.: The interaction of methotrexate and 5-fluorouracil. European Journal of Cancer 9: 733-739 (1973).

Tattersall, M.H.N.; Jackson, R.C.; Jackson, S.T.M. and Harrap, K.R.: Factors determining cell sensitivity to methotrexate. European Journal of Cancer 10: 819-826 (1974).

Thomas, E.D. and Storb, R.: The effect of amethopterin on the immune response. Annals of the New York Academy of Sciences 186: 467-474 (1971).

Ultmann, J.E.: Current status: The management of lymphoma. Seminars in Haematology 7: 441-460 (1970).

Ultmann, J.E. and Nixon, D.D.: The therapy of lymphoma. Seminars in Haematology 6: 376-403 (1969).

Valeriote, F. and Lin, H.: Synergistic interaction of anticancer agents: A cellular perspective. Cancer Chemotherapy Reports 59: 895-900 (1975).

Walker, M.D.: Treatment of brain tumours. Medical Clinics of North America 61: 1045-1051 (1977).

Walters, T.R.: The definitive treatment of children with acute leukaemia. Medical Clinics of North America 60: 987-1000 (1976).

Warwick, O.H.; Darte, J.M.M. and Brown, T.C.: Some biological effects of vincaleukoblastine, an alkaloid in Vinca rosea Linn in patients with malignant disease. Cancer Research 20: 1032-1040 (1960).

Watkins, P.J.; Fairley, G.H. and Scott, R.B.: Treatment of polycythemia. British Medical Journal 2: 664-666 (1967).

Weinstein, G.D.: Biochemical and pathophysiological rationale for amethopterin in psoriasis. Annals of the New York Academy of Sciences 186: 452-466 (1971).

Young, R.C.; Canellos, G.P.; Chabner, B.A.; Schein, P.S. and DeVita, V.T.: Maintenance chemotherapy for advanced Hodgkin's disease in remission. Lancet 2: 1339-1343 (1973).

Young, R.C.; Hubbard, S.P. and DeVita, V.T.: The chemotherapy of ovarian carcinoma. Cancer Treatment Reviews 1: 99-110 (1974).

Ziegler, J.L.: Chemotherapy of Burkitt's lymphoma. Cancer 30: 1534-1540 (1972).

Ziegler, J.L.: Burkitt's lymphoma. Medical Clinics of North America 61: 1073-1082 (1977).

Zubrod, C.G.: The basis for progress in chemotherapy. Cancer 30: 1474-1479 (1972).

Index

H

I

K

L

M

N

O

P

R

S

T

U

V

W